try it!
SUPERFOODS
SUPER FAST

try it!

SUPERFOODS
SUPER FAST

by Michael Van Straten & Barbara Griggs

DK INDIA
Project Editor Arani Sinha
Senior Art Editor Ivy Roy
Art Editor Jomin Johny
Deputy Managing Editor Bushra Ahmed
Managing Art Editor Navidita Thapa
Pre-Production Manager Sunil Sharma
Senior DTP Designer Pushpak Tyagi
DTP Designer Manish Upreti

DK UK
Project Editor Kathryn Meeker
Senior Art Editor Anne Fisher
Managing Editor Stephanie Farrow
Managing Art Editor Christine Keilty
Jacket Designer Amy Keast
Producer, Pre-Production Andy Hilliard
Producer Stephanie McConnell
Creative Technical Support Sonia Charbonnier
Photographer Sïan Irvine

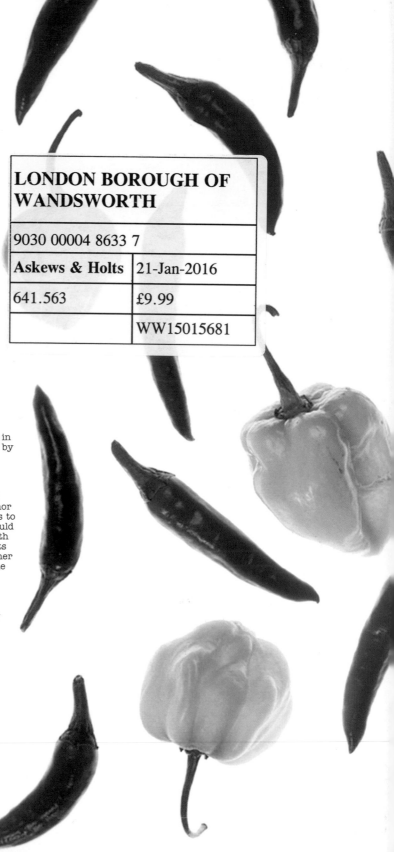

First published in Great Britain in 2016 by
Dorling Kindersley Limited,
80 Strand, London WC2R 0RL

Copyright © 2016 Dorling Kindersley Limited
A Penguin Random House Company
2 4 6 8 10 9 7 5 3 1
001 – 290928– Jan/2016

Some text from the Superfoods section first appeared in
Superfeast by Michael van Straten, published in 2005 by
Little Books, Inc. Text here is reproduced by kind
permission of the publisher.

A CIP catalogue record for this book
is available from the British Library.
ISBN 978-0-2412-4827-0

Printed and bound in China.

All images © Dorling Kindersley Limited
For further information see: www.dkimages.com

A WORLD OF IDEAS:
SEE ALL THERE IS TO KNOW

www.dk.com

Contents

A cookery book with a difference

When we first coined the word "Superfoods" 25 years ago, it was to describe the best of all ordinary, everyday foods with the highest nutritional value for money. Apples, pears, parsnips, turnips, strawberries, blackberries, cherries, pumpkins, cabbage, spinach, nuts and seeds together with all the protein rich dairy products, fish, meat, and poultry.

Now, the supermarkets, the food industry, and even the health food business have jumped on the bandwagon so they can make huge profits by selling the idea of Superfoods as exotic berries and strange products from the other side of the world. These are all high-cost items that you do not need. Spend your money at the market, farm shop, or supermarket on the items in our book and you will get real Superfood value for your money and your health.

The purpose of this book is to help people suffering from specific ailments in the simplest, most effective way – by teaching them to eat and enjoy those foods that will promote the healing process, and to avoid those that aggravate the condition, or indeed, may have caused it in the first place.

Equally, you can use this book to help promote the health and improve the resistance of yourself and your whole family by serving up a daily diet of Superfoods.

Your health problem may be a disabling bout of flu, or a crippling case of arthritis; you may be coping with an annual visitation of bronchitis, or chronic digestive discomfort, or even a diagnosis of cancer.

All of the Superfoods can be found in the first half of the book. Some of them have a centuries-long history of successful kitchen medicine, such as sauerkraut for digestive problems. However, we certainly do not imply that any fruit, or other healthy food not named is without value to you and should be avoided. On the contrary, we always urge that you eat from as wide a range of foodstuffs as possible. So whatever your health problem, choose freely (unless you have been advised by a medical professional to avoid particular foods).

How can you get the most out of this book?

Study the Superfoods to find which might be the most beneficial to you. In the recipe section you'll find dozens of other dishes that feature your Superfoods.

All of the recipes are beneficial for many ailments, but the ailments for which a recipe is most effective are listed under its title. Obviously, you don't have to keep eating the same dishes week after week. However, after using them you may find it easier, and certainly cheaper, to plan a whole week's eating plan in the same way, balancing starch and protein, and including two or three Superfoods at almost every meal.

Super-resistance

In an ideal world, the food we eat would be organically grown in soil uncontaminated by heavy metals and acid rain; the vegetables we eat would be freshly picked from our own gardens; the water we drink would be spring-pure and the air we breathe mountain-fresh. For the vast majority of us, this ideal is as remote as the Garden of Eden.

Our bodies suffer the daily insult of pollutants and the stress of food that is often deficient in micronutrients. The fact that the human race has evolved at all is remarkable. We survive at what cost?

We are seeing today a dramatic increase in chronic diseases such as heart disease, asthma, eczema, depression and Irritable Bowel Disease. Most shocking of all is the world's growing obesity crisis, which will see almost three-quarters of men and two-thirds of women in the UK being overweight by 2030, health experts have said, with similar figures from most Western countries.

Many of these will go on to develop, and have their lives shortened by, diabetes. In the USA, according to 2014 figures, 29.1 million people or 9.3 per cent of the population have diabetes, diagnosed and undiagnosed. In Australia, 280 new cases are diagnosed every day. Similar figures could be quoted for every such chronic condition, and there is no sign of the epidemic slowing.

Many workers in the field of environmental medicine believe that our growing health problems are a consequence of our diet of devitalised foods, the product of agribusiness and global contamination. As early as 1972, a study by the Food and Agriculture

Organization reported severe zinc deficiencies in a wide range of soils in Europe and the United States. Fruit and vegetables grown on depleted soils are often low in vital minerals and trace elements, especially zinc, magnesium, and selenium, and there is no sign of any general improvement in farming methods. In fact, intensive farming today relies on ever-increasing amounts of chemical fertilizer and pesticides that linger in our foodstuffs, further depleting our nutritional reserves.

Today, more than ever, if we want to enjoy vibrant health, we need to eat from a menu rich in natural goodness and freshness. We need a diet of Superfoods, foods with the highest protective value, which will help build our natural resistance, and provide the full spectrum of nutrients our bodies need.

Today it is not enough simply to rely on the traditional well-balanced mixed diet. To ensure Super-resistance, you must know how to supplement your diet – not with pills and capsules, but with the Superfoods that are extra-rich sources of the natural goodness we need. Treat these foods as extra insurance at times of need, whether physical, mental, or emotional; during pregnancy, flu epidemics, periods of overwork or unusually high stress, or after an indulgent holiday. Use them at times of illness to hasten your recovery and always make sure that they feature regularly in your everyday eating. After all, an ounce of prevention really is worth a pound of cure.

Eating healthily doesn't have to cost a fortune. In terms of nutrition, more expensive certainly doesn't mean more valuable. The cheapest shin of beef is no less nutritious than a Chateaubriand steak; and common, locally grown vegetables will actually be fresher and more vitamin-rich than expensive, much-travelled, out-of-season alternatives.

Try to buy as many fresh, unpackaged, unprocessed foods as possible. Not only will they cost much less than pre-packed foods, but they will also be considerably fresher and thus a better buy nutritionally. Befriend your local butcher, greengrocer, and fishmonger. They will be able to advise you on how to cook unfamiliar joints, vegetables, or fish, which may be the cheapest buy of the day. This is even more important if you're shopping just for one person, since many pre-packed foods are designed for a minimum of two people. Get into the habit of planning meals two or three days ahead. Learn to be resourceful with leftovers. Resist the almost irresistible impulse buys, as you push the supermarket trolley between shelves groaning with tempting delights. Most important of all, learn to be creative and experimental in your kitchen. If you do not have every single ingredient in a recipe, you can find a substitute – short of total incineration, you have to do something extremely awful to render food inedible. You will soon discover that you don't have to spend a great deal of money to eat healthily. We costed two sets of menus, buying all of the items at the same snack bars or supermarkets. Eating the healthy Superfood menus actually cost us at least 10 per cent less than the equivalent junk food menus.

In the affluent Western world, an enormous amount of money is spent on junk food. Among the best-selling foods in Britain, cola drinks, white sugar, potato crisps, and chocolate bars are all in the premier league, raking in well over £500 million a year. Nutritionally, such foods contribute almost nothing but calories.

Before you say, "My diet is fine", or "I wouldn't feed my family on that rubbish", keep a notebook for one week and faithfully record every single item of food or drink that goes into your mouth. Get your family to do the same. At the end of the week, add up just how much high-fat, high-sugar, and low-nutrient foods and drinks have come your way. Count every biscuit, sweet, chocolate, fizzy drink, greasy take-away, packet of crisps, ice-cream dessert, bag of chips, pork pie, and sausage roll that you have bought. Then work out how much they've cost you.

The more knowledgeable you are about nutrition, the easier it is to make good choices of food for yourself and your family. It's perfectly true that a burger and French fries, or a helping of the best fish and chips in the neighbourhood, are fun food once in a while and will do you no harm if eaten occasionally. Similarly, everybody likes a bar of chocolate now and then. In a heatwave, what can be more delicious than a good ice cream? However, it is when these foods become part of your staple diet, and when they crowd the good, health-building foods out of your budget, that your health will suffer. This is the price you're paying.

All you'll ever need to know about nutrition

Your great-grandmother may never have heard the word "nutrition". She didn't know a carbohydrate from a protein, a good fat from a bad fat, or a vitamin from a mineral. In spite of this, she raised your grandmother, who raised your mother, who raised you. How on earth did she do it without the help of nutrition experts, with their lists and diagrams? Simple, she used common sense. She served foods that were fresh and in season, and she planned good, square meals with a wide range of ingredients, which the family sat down to and enjoyed together. Nutritionists have been arguing about exactly what we should be eating ever since the first vitamin was discovered in the early years of the last century. Today, however, there is nearly complete agreement throughout the world. The rules of sound nutrition can be summed up quite simply:

★ Eat plenty of fresh fruit and vegetables
★ Eat a large variety of foods
★ Eat more fibre
★ Eat less fat
★ Eat much less sugar
★ Eat less salt

Here is what you need to know about the foods you eat.

VEGETABLES AND FRUIT

For thousands of years, our human ancestors lived on a diet that was largely plant-based, with occasional meat or fish, and eventually grains. It has been calculated that they probably sampled dozens of different plants - nuts, seeds, leaves, roots, fruits - over a year. And since any plant is made up of hundreds of different chemical compounds, the intake of these was huge.

These plant compounds are called Phytochemicals, and growing numbers of those are being identified and studied. We now know that our plant food will supply us with far more than just vitamins, minerals, and trace elements. They provide a whole pharmacy of natural medicines for our needs - anti-inflammatories, diuretics, anti-oxidants, anti-histamines, tonics for the heart and lung, the liver and the digestive system, and protection against cancer.

These phytochemicals are present in infinitesimal amounts in plants, but like individual notes in music, they work together to create complexes of healing for those regularly tucking into the foods, herbs, the spices in which they abound.

Research is proving that a diet high in plant foods is powerfully protective of our health. In 2014, researchers at University College London studied the eating habits of over 65,000 people over 12 years. They found that the more fruit and vegetables they ate, the less likely they were to die at any age. Compared to eating less than a single portion of fruit or vegetables a day, the risk of death by any cause, they calculated, is reduce by 14 per cent for those eating 1-3 portions, 29 per cent for 3-5 portions, 36 per cent for 5-7 portions, and 42 per cent for 7 or more portions.

CARBOHYDRATES

Carbohydrates occur in grains, such as wheat and rice; pulses, such as beans and lentils; and in some root vegetables, such as potatoes, parsnips, and yams. These are often referred to as "complex carbohydrates". All you need to know is that foods such as wholemeal bread, brown rice, certain breakfast cereals (porridge, shredded wheat, unsweetened muesli), pasta, beans, and potatoes, are all wholesome. They are good because they provide slow release energy and a wide range of nutrients. They are generally inexpensive and bulky, and traditional, healthy diets all over the world are based largely on grains and pulses. These "good" carbohydrates tend to have a low GI (glycaemic index) rating. This means they're converted slowly from carbohydrates into sugars without causing a sudden rush of insulin into the bloodstream. Low GI foods protect against diabetes, obesity, bowel cancer, and heart disease.

Confusingly, sugars are also carbohydrates, and these are not good for you, especially if they supply most of the energy in your diet. In fact, sugar is now considered by most researchers to be largely responsible for our epidemic of obesity and diabetes today, especially in the form of sweet fizzy drinks and confectionery. Refined sugars, such as sucrose, glucose, dextrose, and maltose, are used in massive quantities in processed foods, including savoury products, such as baked beans and tomato soup. You can often find three or four of them listed in the ingredients on food packets. These sugars do not need processing by the body and are absorbed straight into the bloodstream, stimulating the pancreas to produce excess insulin. These are high GI foods and excessive consumption may lead to weight gain and a condition called insulin resistance, a forerunner of type 2 diabetes. This condition is known as "adult onset diabetes", as it normally begins in middle age. Tragically, because of the enormous consumption of high GI carbohydrates, doctors are now seeing type 2 diabetes in children as young as eight years old. The sugars that your body produces from low GI carbohydrates do not have this effect.

Grains such as wheat, oats, and barley have for centuries been a staple of diets round the world. Unfortunately, the highly refined wheat and rice we see today are unhealthy foods, and wheat in particular - in modern hybridised versions, baked industrially into the modern sliced wrapped loaf and turning up in dozens of different processed foods - is producing an epidemic of gluten intolerance. If you suspect you may be a sufferer, try eating bread made from the ancient spelt grain used by the Romans, or sourdough bread, made by a primitive and slower method. Until early this century, most of the rice eaten around the world was unpolished, brown rice. What is "refined" out of wheat and rice is most of the goodness. In many countries in the West, including Britain, the United States, Canada, Australia, and New Zealand, certain of these nutrients must by law be added back to the flour before it is baked into bread, but many vital nutrients are not.

FAT
For decades, almost all the "experts" told us that saturated fats - butter, cheese, lard, whole milk, beef, pork - were bad for us, causing cholesterol levels to pile up in our arteries for an epidemic of heart disease. Instead we should eat polyunsaturated fats such as margarine and sunflower oil, and only enjoy dairy in its low-fat forms. It now turns out that the science behind the low-fat commandment was hijacked by the food industry, which crammed its low-fat yoghurts with sugar and other artificial ingredients, and used billions of tons of margarine and sugar in its processed foods.

Today, the advice is enjoy animal fats in moderation. Remember that it's the cream in milk that supplies most of its nutritional value. You need to know, too, that the type of fat we are most likely to be short of is what are known as the omega-3 fats, found in oily fish like salmon and sardines, and in walnuts, hazelnuts, and the germ of wheat that's lost in refining. Most polyunsaturated margarine is a highly processed, unnatural foodstuff that contains

trans-fatty acids. These trans-fats are liquid fats that are chemically treated to make them solid at room temperature, and they appear to be decidedly unhealthy. Natural butter, on the other hand, if used in moderation, is a useful source of vitamins A, D, and E.

We now know what every Mediterranean peasant has always known - that extra-virgin olive oil is a wonderful foundation on which to build your daily diet and it is the best oil for your health, especially if it is combined with plenty of garlic and a glass of red wine a day. This is hardly surprising. Extra-virgin olive oil is obtained by a simple pressure process and contains the natural goodness found in the olive. The consumption of vegetable oils (such as sunflower, safflower, and corn oil) for cooking has rocketed this century. Many of them are heavily processed to turn them into the near tasteless products you buy. Consequently, there is little of the natural goodness of the sunflower, the safflower, or the corn left in them and they have an unhealthy ratio of omega-6 to omega-3 fats.

With Superfoods, your diet will not be high in fat. Consequently, you can enjoy the pleasures of real butter, the occasional dollop of cream, and proper whole milk - instead of skimmed milk, which is nutritionally a poor second cousin to the real thing and should never be given to children under age five. Full fat milk only contains 4 per cent fat, which means it could legally be labelled as a low fat food.

PROTEIN
Estimates of how much protein - body-building components - we need to keep us going have varied wildly, from the hefty 150g (5oz) a day proposed by 19th-century nutritionists (equivalent to the protein content of approximately 600g/1lb of lean beef) to the more modest 55-90g (2-3oz) for adults that is recommended today.

How do you know whether you're getting enough protein? Simple. Unless you are following an extreme form of diet, such as a food-exclusion diet, or you are an exceptionally faddy eater or an anorexic, it is almost impossible to be protein-deficient on an average, mixed diet. Quite the reverse is true. If you are eating eggs and bacon for breakfast, a pork pie at lunchtime, and meat and two vegetables in the evening, you may well be consuming far more protein than your body needs and your kidneys will feel the strain. Furthermore, meat isn't the only good source of protein, as is obvious when you consider the world's millions of healthy vegetarians. For those with high blood pressure, it is useful to know that reducing your animal protein intake helps to bring it down. Fish, chicken, eggs, cheese, milk, beans, peas, nuts, grains, vegetables, and even some fruits all supply varying quantities of protein. The average Western adult gets around 66 per cent of his or her protein from meat, fish, eggs, cheese, and milk; 25 per cent from bread and other cereals; and 10 per cent from vegetables.

In spite of many doctors' opposition to vegetarianism, some of the healthiest cultures in the world never eat meat or animal products. The wisdom of centuries-old eating traditions helps these peoples balance their diets without even thinking about it. The old idea of first-class and second-class proteins, with meat belonging in the executive class, is now, thankfully, dying out. The only imperative for vegetarians is that they should get their protein from mixed sources, as in the traditional rice and peas of the West Indies, for example; the rice and lentils of the Middle East; the pasta and beans of Italy; and the rice and dhal of India.

However, it is virtually impossible to be an adult vegan – someone who avoids eggs and all milk products as well as meat and fish – without supplementing the diet with B vitamins. It is risky to bring up a child as a vegan unless you are extremely well-informed and give the child the appropriate dietary supplements.

FIBRE

Fibre occurs in whole grains, pulses, vegetables, fruits, and seeds. A hundred years ago nobody needed to worry about fibre, since it was naturally present in their daily bread, cereals, and vegetables. There is now a huge body of evidence to suggest that when your diet is deficient in fibre, you are likely to suffer from a whole range of digestive nasties. As well as benefiting the digestive system, certain forms of fibre, especially the type in oats, barley, and beans, help the body eliminate excess cholesterol, and consequently protect the heart and circulatory system. And there's another, more urgent, reason for upping your intake of fibre. We now know that the trillions of micro-organisms that live mainly in our gut, but also in every other part of our bodies, are crucially important to our general health and well-being. They need plenty of vegetable fibre to keep them thriving - particularly the type called inulin found in high amounts in garlic and leeks.

VITAMINS AND MINERALS

Even a qualified nutritionist would need a computer to work out how many of your daily vitamin and mineral needs will be met by a particular diet or food.

Without burdening you with an incomprehensible array of numbers, here are some simple guidelines to ensure that you obtain all of your vitamin and mineral requirements from the food you eat.

★ The fresher the fruit and vegetables you eat, the better they are for you. Much of their goodness starts to disappear the moment they are picked. The loss of vitamin C is increased by storage, handling, bruising, and preparation. Heat is the final enemy of vitamin C. The most nutritious way of eating many vegetables and most fruit is raw. Try one meal a day of nothing but raw foods – wonderful fruit, delicious salads, a crunchy carrot or cauliflower, peppers, fennel, celery, and unroasted nuts. Keeping cooked vegetables warm will destroy what little vitamin C may be left. B vitamins and many minerals leach out into the cooking water, so cook vegetables in a minimum of water, for the shortest possible time.

★ Good, fresh produce is always the first choice when it comes to buying vegetables. Commercially frozen vegetables are also a good option, since they are harvested and frozen at their best, when their vitamin content is at its highest. They may lose some vitamin C, but they will contain more than vegetables that have spent a long time in transit, in the shop, or in your vegetable rack. Frozen vegetables are handy for the cook who is pressed for time, since they can turn a snack into a nutritious meal.

★ Discover nuts and seeds – they're not just for the budgie. Almonds, hazelnuts, walnuts, cashews, and chestnuts, and sunflower, sesame, and pumpkin seeds are all available in supermarkets, and they're delicious. They also happen to be bursting with B vitamins, vitamin E, zinc, iron, protein, and fibre – the nutrients for their future growth into trees, shrubs, and flowers.

★ There are super-nutrients and anti-nutrients. All the vitamins are essential for life, but some are super-nutrients, such as beta-carotene, which is found in brightly coloured fruits and vegetables and is converted by the body into vitamin A. Vitamin C from fresh produce and vitamin E from nuts and seeds are also super-nutrients. Some super-nutrients are antioxidants that mop up excess free radicals, which are the by-products of body chemistry. These are highly destructive to individual cells, and they can trigger cancer, heart disease, and other disorders. Free radicals are also responsible for visible signs of aging, such as wrinkles.

An ever-growing body of research has now established beyond doubt the key role of antioxidants in keeping us healthy. Eat plenty of green leaves, red peppers, grated carrot, radishes, fennel, chopped parsley, and tomatoes, dressed with extra-virgin olive oil, and you'll be enjoying a mega-helping of the antioxidants.

Anti-nutrients are substances that either interfere with the body's absorption of nutrients or destroy them. The much-touted bran, lavishly packed into cereals, or sprinkled into soup, can have a disastrous effect on the absorption of calcium, iron, and other minerals. Drunk at mealtimes, coffee, tea, and other caffeine-carriers, such as cola drinks and chocolate, can lower the amount of iron that the body will absorb from food. Vitamin C, on the other hand, will maximize it, so if you must have coffee with your boiled egg (a good source of iron), have some orange juice with it as well.

Refined sugars and alcohol drain the body's vitamin B reserves. Certain drugs also lower nutrient uptake or bodily stores of nutrients, among them antibiotics, the contraceptive pill, antidepressants, antacids, and laxatives. If you are taking any of these regularly, your diet should be especially good and you should consider taking a simple vitamin supplement.

★ At least once a day, eat a home-cooked meal (at the table, not in front of the television), and not in a rush. This way of eating is good for your digestion and results in your body getting more nutrients from the food. This is not to mention the fact that you and your partner, your family, or your friends will gather around the table and talk to one another, something that few people make time to do these days.

If you can't manage a daily gathering around the dining table, why not try resurrecting the traditional Sunday lunch, or making a Friday evening family feast part of your weekly routine? Such gatherings are often among our richest childhood memories, but how many of today's children will be able to look back on them?

How carefully should you stick to the Superfoods?

If you are seriously or chronically ill, if a doctor or specialist has recently given you a diagnosis of bad news, the more you build the appropriate Superfoods into your daily menu, the more dramatic will be the improvement in your condition, and the sooner you may return to health. Superfoods cannot guarantee full recovery, but they can always help reduce painful

symptoms and increase well-being. In our present state of ignorance, it would be foolhardy and irresponsible to claim that dietary changes alone can produce cures, but there can be no doubt that the right food will maximize the body's ability to fight back against many diseases. The extraordinary healing power of nature operates best in the well nourished organism, whether it is a single cell or a complex human being.

Recent studies show the importance of nutritional factors in the amelioration of many diseases. For this reason we would urge all sufferers from such conditions as AIDS, myalgic encephalopathy (ME), Parkinson's disease, Alzheimer's disease, multiple sclerosis, motor neurone disease, cancer, lupus, rheumatoid arthritis, epilepsy, and schizophrenia to contact the relevant self-help and research organizations for the most up to date information and advice.

Pick the recipes that take your fancy, enjoy them, and know that every mouthful enhances your health. As doctors are at last beginning to acknowledge, nature heals. However, *Superfoods Super Fast* was designed to maintain well-being, as well as help restore it, and you certainly don't need to be ill or out of condition to enjoy and benefit from the recipes in this book.

It's a good idea to make a list of your personal Superfoods. By the time you've been consulting it for a few days, you'll probably end up knowing it by heart. Then when you eat out in a restaurant, canteen, or café, you'll be able to skim the menu and tell at a glance which are the good choices and which should be off-limits.

You can have too much of a good thing, even of a Superfood. Some of these foods can be used successfully in what is known as the mono-fast – when you eat nothing but apples, or grapes, or plain brown rice for a day or two to help cleanse and regenerate your bodily forces – but few foods are suitable for such frequent consumption. Even ordinary and everyday foods, such as carrots, wholewheat bread, and oranges, should not be overeaten. Some foods, such as pineapples or strawberries, can actually be harmful if eaten to excess. Let common sense be your guide. Eat the Superfoods that are right for you. Eat them often. Eat them daily, but don't overdo it.

The Superfoods

* ★ Fruit
* ★ Vegetables
* ★ Grains and pulses
* ★ Nuts and seeds
* ★ Eggs and dairy
* ★ Meat, seafood, and poultry
* ★ Herbs and spices
* ★ Miscellaneous

Apples

★★★★

"If you could plant only one tree in your garden, it should be an apple tree", says famous French herbalist Maurice Messegue. So what's in an apple? A bonus for your heart: the pectin and vitamin C in apples help keep cholesterol levels stable, as US studies have shown; pectin also protects us from the ravages of pollution, binding to heavy metals, such as lead or mercury, in the body and carrying them safely out. The malic and tartaric acids in apples help to neutralize the acid by-products of indigestion and help your body cope with excess protein or rich, fatty foods: apple purée with pork, apples with cheese, or sage and apple stuffing for goose are traditional combinations based on country wisdom.

Because of these qualities, these wonderful autumn fruits are great detoxifiers, and people suffering from arthritis, rheumatism, or gout should eat raw apples regularly. A mono-fast on apples alone, for a day or two, can be warmly recommended for people suffering from food poisoning or inflammatory bowel conditions. It's also a marvellous general pick-me-up after the excesses of a holiday or festive season, or a debilitating bout of flu.

It was observation of an apple cure at work that led Dr Bircher-Benner to his discovery of the healing powers of raw food. On the advice of an old doctor, he fed grated raw apple to a patient whose digestive problems had brought her close to death: it was the first food she was able to take in weeks, and after a few days of the apple cure, she was well on the way to recovery. Apples, as Bircher-Benner realized, are first-class therapy for any digestive problems or infections, being both soothing and antiseptic.

In a French study, eating two apples a day resulted in an average drop in cholesterol levels of up to 10 per cent. That's partly because apples are also a fantastic source of fibre, both soluble and insoluble: one large apple can provide 10 per cent of your daily recommended fibre intake. And we now know that high-fibre foods can be useful in preventing heart disease.

Recommended for:
circulatory
digestive
joints

Pears

★★★★

Pears are a good source of pectin, which helps bowel function and increases the amount of cholesterol eliminated by the body. Supplying reasonable vitamin C, some vitamin A and E, and potassium, they're helpful for digestion and convalescence, and are a source of easily accessible good calories. They contain no fat and virtually no sodium, but they do contain fruit sugar, which is easily converted into instantly usable energy.

Pears are one of the foods least likely to cause any type of allergic reaction, so they're ideal puréed for babies and used in exclusion diets where food allergies or intolerances are suspected. However, fresh pears do contain a sugar-based alcohol called sorbitol. While this sugar-free sweetener is tooth-friendly, in large amounts it may cause diarrhoea in a small number of susceptible people.

Recommended for:
circulatory
digestive

Oranges

★★★★

The high vitamin C content of fresh oranges accounts for much of their beneficial influence on our health, given the vital importance of this vitamin in combating infection. Here's one more bonus: in a Swedish study of people eating a Western-style breakfast, orange juice taken at the same meal more than doubled iron absorption. Oranges also contain another antioxidant: the vitamin A precursor beta-carotene.

The pith and segment walls contain bioflavonoids. These are also known as vitamin P factors, or C2 since they appear to make possible the activity of vitamin C. In addition they are known to strengthen the walls of the capillaries. Leslie Kenton points out that in the original plant, these compounds "act as primitive defence systems protecting them from disease...Many studies indicate that various bioflavonoids...actively combat infectious bacteria, viruses and fungi."

• • • • • • • • • • • • • • • • •

Recommended for:
cancer
circulatory
respiratory
skin

Grapefruit

★★★★

Grapefruit shares with other citrus fruits a high level of vitamin C and plenty of potassium. It's also well supplied with pectin – a substance recommended to those suffering from circulatory or digestive problems. In addition, grapefruit has high concentrations of bioflavonoids. These plant substances are attracting increasing medical interest. They seem to have the ability to protect the integrity of the blood vessels, particularly the tiny capillaries, and to act against inflammation. Both pectin and bioflavonoids are found in the white pith of grapefruit, and in the membranes dividing the sections, so eat the whole fruit rather than just the juice to ensure maximum benefit.

• • • • • • • • • • • • • • • • • • •

Recommended for:
circulatory
digestive
respiratory

Lemons and limes

★★★★

Limes are the most acid of citrus fruits, containing more vitamin C than grapefruit but less than oranges and lemons. Mostly grown for juice used as flavouring, particularly in drinks, limes have a similar chemical composition and medicinal properties to lemon juice. They're also rich in protective bioflavonoids, which are found mostly in the pith.

Royal Navy ships carried barrels of limes to prevent scurvy. This is the origin of the epithet "limey", an American name for an English person.

● ● ● ● ● ● ● ● ● ● ● ● ● ● ● ● ● ● ●

Recommended for:
cancer
respiratory

Blueberries

★★★★

Blueberries were introduced to early settlers in North America by the Native Americans, for whom they were a staple food. Along with cranberries, the high vitamin C content in blueberries prevented them from dying of scurvy. The pigment, which is mostly in the skin, has a high concentration of antioxidants. Blueberries may even help to prevent Alzheimer's disease and other forms of dementia. Containing more antioxidant chemicals than red wine, blueberries are good for the heart and circulation. Added to breakfast smoothies or sprinkled over your morning cereal, they are a powerful package.

Recommended for:
cancer
circulatory
digestive
stress

Cranberries

★★★★

The Native Americans taught white settlers in North America to eat the tart, bright red berries of the cranberry bush as a remedy for scurvy, and Yankee ships soon routinely carried barrels of cranberries stored in water. The berries are high in vitamin C; but iron, vitamin A, and potassium are among their other nutritional assets.

Worldwide, scientists now accept what Native American medicine men have always known – that cranberry juice both treats and prevents urinary tract infections. It's not the acidity of the cranberries that does the trick, but their natural mucilage, which sticks to the walls of the bladder and its associated structures. This mucilage prevents bacteria from lodging in the tissues and causing chronic and recurrent cystitis. In a number of trials, cranberry juice has been used to treat urinary tract infections over prolonged periods with no marked side effects. There's no evidence of bacterial resistance to the benefits of this amazing juice.

• • • • • • • • • • • • • • • • • • •

Recommended for:
circulatory
fatigue
urinary

Raspberries
★★★★

Like grapes, raspberries should be on every hospital menu. This tart, delectable fruit supplies not only a fair amount of vitamin C, but useful amounts of calcium, potassium, iron, and magnesium, which are all vital to the convalescent, as well as to those suffering from heart problems, fatigue, or depression. All of the minerals are well absorbed, thanks to the vitamin C.

Herbalists value raspberries for their cooling effect – they are useful in feverish conditions. Naturally astringent, raspberries can do you good the length of your digestive tract, helping to counter spongy, diseased gums, upset stomachs, and diarrhoea along the way.

· · · · · · · · · · · · · · · · ·

Recommended for:
circulatory
digestive
stress

Strawberries

★ ★ ★ ★

The great Swedish botanist Linnaeus, whose special interest was in medicinal plants, recommended strawberries as a perfect cure for arthritis, gout, and rheumatism. He spoke from personal experience: he cured himself of gout by eating almost nothing but strawberries morning and night. This agreeable cure probably works because strawberries are admirable cleansers and purifiers of the whole system.

Strawberries also have a confirmed reputation for combating high blood pressure, and they are recommended in European traditional medicine for the elimination of kidney stones. Their high iron content makes them therapeutic for anaemia and fatigue. People with skin problems should enjoy plenty of this wonderful fruit, which cleanses and regenerates the intestinal flora. For full therapeutic effect, strawberries should be eaten on their own, or at the start of a meal.

● ● ● ● ● ● ● ● ● ● ● ● ● ● ● ● ● ● ●

Recommended for:
circulatory
fatigue
joints
skin

Apricots

★★★★

Apricots, an early summer fruit that originated in China, are loaded with beta-carotene, as their wonderful yellow-orange colour informs us – the brighter the colour, the more beta-carotene a fruit contains. Beta-carotene – a nutrient which is converted by your body in to vitamin A – is one of the most effective antioxidants around, so the ripe, fresh fruit should be eaten whenever possible by those suffering from any infection (especially of the respiratory system) or at risk from cancer or heart disease.

A US study also found that women who had high vitamin A intakes nearly halved their chances of developing cataracts: the more fruit you eat, the better your eyes. Dried apricots supply iron, and they actually have higher antioxidant levels than the fresh fruit. They can be thrown into stews or added to muesli. The sulphur dioxide that preserves their colour can easily be washed off in some warm water.

Recommended for:
cancer
respiratory
skin

Cherries

★★★★

Cherries contain plenty of potassium and virtually no sodium, so they're excellent for anyone with high blood pressure or heart disease. They're a reasonable source of vitamin C, but they also contain significant amounts of bioflavonoids and other plant chemicals. This puts them pretty near the top of the list of protective antioxidant foods. Their ellagic acid content adds extra value to their anti-cancer properties.

In folk medicine, cherries have long been used for the relief of arthritis and gout. In addition, dried cherry stones make the most wonderful hot bag for muscular pain, joint disorders, and stomach ache. Although there is no scientific evidence for their effectiveness, the anecdotal stories are legion – and even if cherries don't help, they can't hurt. They taste delicious raw, cooked, juiced, or dried. Of the sour cherries, Morello are wonderful for cooking and Acerola the richest in nutrients.

● ● ● ● ● ● ● ● ● ● ● ● ● ● ● ● ● ●

Recommended for:
cancer
circulatory
joints

Grapes

A bunch of grapes is the present that kind people take to their sick friends in hospital: they could do nothing better for them. Grapes are a uniquely nourishing, strengthening, cleansing, and regenerative food, useful in convalescence.

Grapes are also excellent for easing the symptoms of anaemia, fatigue, and disorders such as arthritis, gout, and rheumatism, that may result from poor elimination of waste products, such as urine. The nutritive powers of grapes were confirmed by Mahatma Gandhi, who drank grape juice during his marathon fasts.

In 1926 South African natural healer Johanna Brandt pioneered the grape cure, after claiming to have cured herself of cancer with its help: for weeks on end, she ate nothing but fresh grapes. European nature clinics have obtained excellent results using a grape mono-fast to treat a range of ailments, including skin problems, disorders of the urinary system, arthritis, and gout. A two-day grape mono-fast every ten days is recommended for those wanting to lose weight.

Grapes should be eaten on their own, and not as part of a meal. This is because they ferment rapidly in the stomach. Chewing grapes is also recommended to help alleviate infected gums.

Grapeseed oil, now increasingly seen on supermarket shelves, is rich in polyunsaturated fats and vitamin E. It's also highly heat stable, even in prolonged cooking at modest temperatures.

It is important to note that most grapes are sprayed incessantly with pesticides during cultivation. Bearing this in mind, it is vital that you wash grapes very carefully indeed before eating them.

. . . .

Recommended for:
cancer
stress
fatigue
joints
skin
urinary

Kiwifruit

★★★★

Kiwifruit isn't just a pretty face in a nouvelle cuisine dish. This little fruit with the shabby fur coat is a treasury of nutritional riches. It contains almost twice as much vitamin C as oranges, more fibre than apples, and as much vitamin E as an avocado – about 3.5mg per 100g (3½oz) serving.

Kiwifruit is particularly rich in potassium, which can be in dangerously short supply in Western diets. Deficiency can lead to high blood pressure, depression, fatigue, and poor digestion. The average kiwifruit will supply 250mg potassium, but only 4mg sodium.

Kiwifruit is often bargain-priced in markets – choose fruit soft enough to yield to gentle pressure. It can be stored in the fridge, and should be peeled just before eating. The nicest way to eat it is like a boiled egg – cut off the top and scoop out the wonderful pale green flesh with its small black seeds.

• • • • • • • • • • • • • • • • • • •

Recommended for:
circulatory
digestive
stress
skin

Bananas

★★★★

One of Nature's most superb fast foods, bananas are unjustly maligned as a high-calorie food; in fact, the average banana contains under 100 calories. Bananas are packed with nourishment, particularly potassium, which is essential to the functioning of every single cell in our bodies. Zinc, iron, folic acid, and calcium are other nutrients that bananas contain. They also contain the useful form of fibre known as pectin, which helps the body to eliminate toxic wastes.

Weight for weight, bananas contain nearly the same amount of vitamin B6 as liver. This important nutrient is chronically undersupplied in the average diet. Bananas are also highly beneficial to the digestive tract, soothing and helping to restore normal function; naturopaths recommend them for both constipation and diarrhoea. They make an ideal energy snack for sporty people, since the potassium helps to prevent cramps. Bananas should be eaten ripe, when they can be easily digested.

• •

Recommended for:
circulatory
digestive
fatigue

Melon

★★★★

Melons are a cooling, delicious treat in hot weather: a large slice of crunchy pink watermelon – sold from roadside stands all over the Mediterranean – beats any canned fizzy drink for refreshment. Watermelon – or a tea made by simmering its seeds in water for 30 minutes – has long been recommended in traditional medicine as a remedy for kidney and bladder problems. All forms of melon are also mildly stimulating to the kidneys, and are gently laxative, making them useful for those with gout or constipation. A two-day mono-fast on melons of any kind is a delightful summer cleanout of the whole system. Like grapes, melon of all kinds should be eaten on its own, or at least at the start of a meal, since it ferments rapidly in the stomach.

• •

Recommended for:
digestive
skin
urinary

Papayas

★★★★

Papaya contains the enzyme papain, which improves digestion. One fruit provides twice the vitamin C and one-third of the vitamin A you need daily. The medicine men of the South American Mayans used the fruit's sticky latex, its juice, and the flesh as medicine. It's still common today in South America to wrap meat in the leaves of the papaya before cooking to create tender and delectable dishes.

On a less culinary note, the leaves may also be used to improve wound healing and for the treatment of leg ulcers and boils in traditional medicine. Even the seeds of this remarkable fruit are useful. The next time you eat a papaya, try saving the seeds and adding them to olive oil, vinegar, or pickles to impart a unique spicy flavour.

Papayas are particularly good for children because they make great-tasting smoothies. Halve and deseed the fruit, put the flesh into a liquidizer, add a small carton of yoghurt and a cup of milk, and whiz until smooth. For a more sophisticated version for adults, whiz the flesh with a little water and mix half and half with champagne.

Although tinned papaya is widely available, it's not nearly as good for you as the fresh fruit, since most of the vitamin C and more than half the beta-carotene are unfortunately lost in processing.

• •

Recommended for:
digestive
respiratory
skin

Mangos

★★★★

One mango provides over a day's dose of vitamin C, two-thirds the recommended amount of vitamin A, nearly half the recommended amount of vitamin E, and a quarter of your fibre, potassium, iron, and nicotinic acid for the day. It also tastes wonderful. Mangos originally grew in India, where their history goes back over 4000 years. Today, varieties are also grown in Australia, South Africa, Brazil, and Pakistan.

It's a fantastic bonus that anything tasting as good as a mango is also a source of powerful antioxidants. The mango also has medicinal properties, and in traditional Indian medicine its antiseptic twigs are chewed to protect the teeth and gums from disease. The bark is used in treating diarrhoea, while the fruit is given for high blood pressure.

Mangos actually belong to the same family as poison ivy. Wear rubber gloves to prepare them to avoid contact with their potentially irritating skin.

• • • • • • • • • • • • • • • • • • • •

Recommended for:
circulatory
fatigue

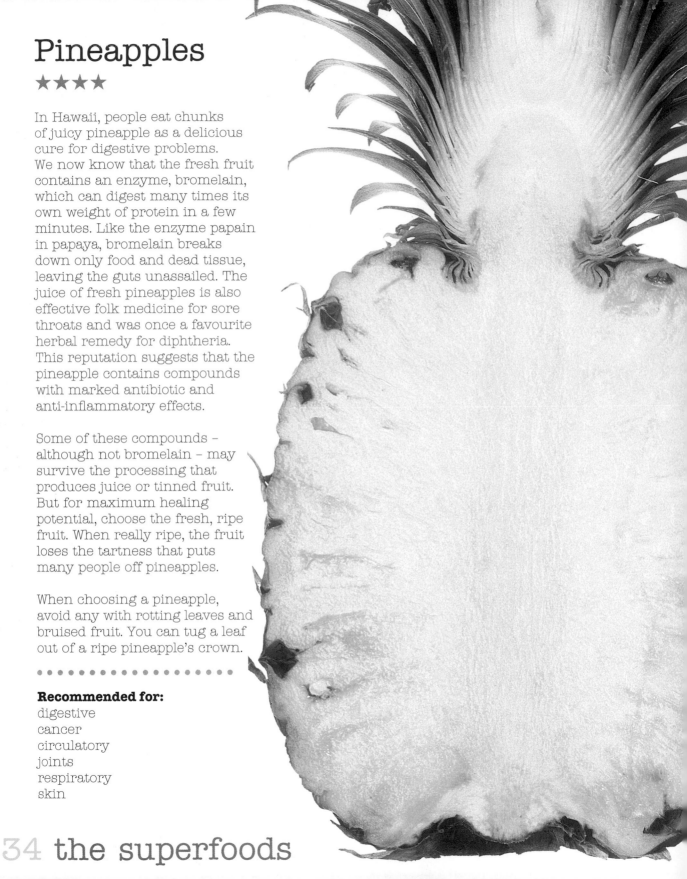

Pineapples
★★★★

In Hawaii, people eat chunks of juicy pineapple as a delicious cure for digestive problems. We now know that the fresh fruit contains an enzyme, bromelain, which can digest many times its own weight of protein in a few minutes. Like the enzyme papain in papaya, bromelain breaks down only food and dead tissue, leaving the guts unassailed. The juice of fresh pineapples is also effective folk medicine for sore throats and was once a favourite herbal remedy for diphtheria. This reputation suggests that the pineapple contains compounds with marked antibiotic and anti-inflammatory effects.

Some of these compounds – although not bromelain – may survive the processing that produces juice or tinned fruit. But for maximum healing potential, choose the fresh, ripe fruit. When really ripe, the fruit loses the tartness that puts many people off pineapples.

When choosing a pineapple, avoid any with rotting leaves and bruised fruit. You can tug a leaf out of a ripe pineapple's crown.

Recommended for:
digestive
cancer
circulatory
joints
respiratory
skin

Pomegranates

★★★★

Pomegranates have been grown and eaten by humans since prehistoric times. This unique fruit has been part of ancient mythology, art, and religion from the time of the ancient Egyptians to the ancient Greeks and the Old Testament. You'll even see it in the mosaic tiles in the excavations at Pompeii. It gets its name from medieval French and it means, literally, "seeded apple" – an average fruit can contain up to 800 of the tiny seeds. Although it has a long history, scientific research shows that the pomegranate is indeed a true Superfood for our modern times.

Scientists in California and Israel have shown that pomegranates are an extraordinarily powerful and natural antioxidant. One small glass of pomegranate juice provides three times the ORAC (Oxygen Radical Absorbance Capacity, a measure of a food's protective qualities) of the same quantity of red wine. What's more, the concentration of protective bioflavonoids in the fruit is even greater than that found in grapes or green tea. All the evidence supports the traditional belief that pomegranates are protective against heart disease, circulatory disorders, degenerative and inflammatory conditions, and even some types of cancer. There are even suggestions that the fruit has antiviral and antibacterial properties. Low in calories, fat, and sodium, pomegranates taste great when freshly juiced.

• •

Recommended for:
cancer
circulatory

Dates

★★★★

Dates are a highly energizing and richly nourishing food that is useful for convalescents and also an excellent addition to packed lunches. They are native to North Africa and Arabia (the date palm is mentioned in the Qur'an more often than any other fruit-bearing plant), and Bedouin Arabs would travel for days across the desert with little more than a store of dates, figs, and flour with which to make unleavened bread.

Like most dried fruits, dates are a good source of the antioxidants that help boost the body's defences against some cancers. Rich in fibre, they are mildly laxative and so prevent constipation. Dates are an important source of minerals and are particularly high in potassium, helping to maintain fluid levels and the sodium/potassium balance so important in very hot climates. Most dates contain easily available iron, but some varieties provide exceptional amounts, which may explain their historical reputation as an aphrodisiac.

● ● ● ● ● ● ● ● ● ● ● ● ● ● ● ● ●

Recommended for:
digestive
respiratory

Figs

★★★★

Figs have a centuries-old reputation as a sustaining and nourishing food. In classical antiquity, athletes were often fed entirely on figs, while Pliny the Elder praised them for their ability to get rid of wrinkles. In either fresh or dried form, they are friendly to the digestion. This is because they contain an enzyme called ficin that assists the digestive process, exerting a soothing action on the gut. They are also mildly laxative. Dried figs are a rich source of fibre, iron, potassium, and calcium, making them a useful food for people with high blood pressure.

Weight for weight, figs contain more fibre than most other fruits or vegetables, so they're great for your digestive system and your cholesterol levels. They're also very high in polyphenol antioxidants, which makes them a valuable food for cancer prevention. The instant energy they provide and their ability to prevent cramps make them good for athletes too.

• • • • • • • • • • • • • • • • • •

Recommended for:
circulatory
digestive
respiratory

the superfoods

Raisins

★★★★

Man has been drying fruits in the sun as a means of preservation for at least 5000 years, and the Romans in particular included raisins in many of their medical prescriptions. Raisins are a perfect energy food for active people and those suffering from exhaustion. They're rich in fibre to help reduce cholesterol and improve bowel function, and also in iron, with a large handful providing more than 25 per cent of the RDA of this nutrient for women. They also contain selenium and potassium, which helps to prevent fluid retention and reduce blood pressure. Raisins contain small amounts of vitamins A and B. The combination of energy and B vitamins means they are helpful for anyone with depression, anxiety, and stress.

Raisins are treated with sulphur or mineral oil, which can both be removed by washing raisins in warm running water. Organic raisins aren't treated with these substances.

• •

Recommended for:
circulatory
stress
fatigue

Prunes

★ ★ ★ ★

These wonderful dried fruits have a terrible reputation. In countries where good food is greatly appreciated, such as France, they're considered a delicacy, whereas we tend to consider them for one thing only – as a laxative – and that's the least of their value. Rich in potassium, which helps high blood pressure, and in fibre, iron, niacin, and vitamins B6 and A, prunes are also energy food. In addition, they also contain *hydroxyphenyl-isatin*, which is a gentle, non-purging laxative. Most importantly, weight for weight, prunes are the most powerful of all the protective antioxidant foods. The US Department of Agriculture has calculated the ORAC (Oxygen Radical Absorbance Capacity) of prunes at 5770 units per 100g (3½oz), compared with 2000-odd for raisins, blueberries, and blackberries. One handful of prunes provides more than the optimum protection of 5000 ORACS daily.

• • • • • • • • • • • • • • • •

Recommended for:
cancer
circulatory
digestive
fatigue

39

Mushrooms

★★★★

We should all eat more mushrooms. They contain more protein than most other vegetables, they're very low in calories, and they're also a good source of phosphorus and potassium. Although most textbooks state that mushrooms are not a source of vitamin B12, the most up-to-date research reveals they are actually a valuable source of this essential nutrient. One decent-sized field mushroom, or three button mushrooms, will give you enough B12 for a day, which is vital for vegetarians and even more so for vegans, as other plant sources of B12 are very limited. The same is true for vitamin E. Again, modern research reveals that most mushrooms are a rich source of this essential nutrient, with 100g (3½oz) providing more than the minimum daily requirement.

Washing spoils their delicate flesh, so just remove any grit from mushrooms and then wipe them clean with a damp cloth.

• • • • • • • • • • • • • • • • • •

Recommended for:
stress
fatigue

Celery

★★★★

Celery helps calm the nerves, according to Hippocrates. Perhaps this is due to its rich calcium content. Worldwide, it has a high reputation as an anti-rheumatic, although the anti-inflammatory agent at the basis of this reputation is more concentrated in the seeds and leaves than in the edible root. In traditional medicine, it's the seeds that are specifically recommended in the form of a tea for gout, rheumatism, and other problems resulting from poor elimination of wastes. In Japan, rheumatic patients are sometimes put on a celery-only diet; celery stewed with milk and eaten with it, or with celery seed tea, is a standard Romany treatment for rheumatic ailments. If you have rheumatoid arthritis, a daily half-glass of celery juice, first thing in the morning, for 15-20 days is worth trying. More than this would be counter-productive, and the kidneys would be irritated rather than stimulated.

As well as these admirable properties, celery has a very high reputation in folk medicine as a sexual stimulant: according to Dr Vogel, it does in fact stimulate not only the thyroid and pituitary glands but also the gonads. There seems little scientific evidence in support of this claim, but folk medicine is seldom wholly misguided. And it's really true – you burn more calories chewing it than you get from eating it.

Recommended for:
digestive
stress
joints
urinary

Radishes

★★★★

Radishes belong to the crucifer family and are valuable for those at risk from cancer. But it is for problems of the liver and gallbladder that traditional medicine has most warmly recommended them. Radish juice acts powerfully on the gallbladder, stimulating the discharge of bile, as French studies have demonstrated.

Radishes contain other nutrients, including plenty of potassium, calcium, and sulphur, as well as some vitamin A and B-complex. They should be eaten as fresh as possible, while still young and crisp. Their tops should be eaten at the same time, as this aids the digestion of the vegetable. However, beware of overindulging in radishes; too much hot, stinging radish can irritate rather than stimulate the liver, kidneys, and gallbladder.

● ● ● ● ● ● ● ● ● ● ● ● ● ● ● ● ● ●

Recommended for:
cancer
digestive
respiratory

Watercress

★★★★

Watercress belongs to the powerful crucifer family, other members of which are cabbage, broccoli, Brussels sprouts, kale, turnip, and radishes. Like them, it should figure prominently in the diet of anyone at risk from cancer. Watercress is also rich in vitamin A and vitamin C, both of which play an important role in combating cancer.

Watercress is related to nasturtiums, and both contain potassium and a benzyl mustard oil, the compound that gives them "bite" and which research has shown to be powerfully antibiotic. Unlike conventional antibiotics, the substances in watercress and nasturtiums are not only harmless to our intestinal flora, they are positively beneficial to the health of our gut. Urinary and respiratory infections in particular benefit from doses of watercress. Watercress is also a good source of iodine, which is useful for those with low thyroid activity.

● ● ● ● ● ● ● ● ● ● ● ● ● ● ● ● ● ●

Recommended for:
cancer
fatigue
respiratory
skin
urinary

Avocados

★★★★

Every slimmer thinks that luscious avocados are a high-fat, high-calorie treat. But when ripe they are also an almost complete food, supplying lots of potassium, vitamins A and E, some B and C vitamins, and a little protein and starch, along with avocado oil, which is mainly a monounsaturated fat.

Avocado is excellent as an early weaning food when puréed with other vegetables, and for convalescents. It's good for anyone suffering from stress or sexual problems. Avocados are a particularly rich source of skin-protective antioxidants, especially vitamin E. Women, in particular, who are often warned off avocados as being extra-high in fat and calories, should eat plenty of this fruit for the sake of their skin. Together with heart-protective monounsaturated oil and the other nutrients they contain, they neutralize damaging free radicals. This makes them good for the heart, circulation, and anti-aging.

• • • • • • • • • • • • • • • • • • •

Recommended for:
circulatory
stress
fatigue
skin

Peppers

★★★★

Known as sweet or bell peppers, these versatile vegetables are an excellent source of vitamin C. The red and yellow ones contain four times as much vitamin C as oranges, and a serving of green peppers will supply 100mg of vitamin C – over three times the recommended daily allowance. For this reason peppers are best eaten raw, although in the salad form popular in Spain or Italy, they conserve much of their vitamin C. Yellow and orange peppers are also a good source of beta-carotene, and of iron and potassium too. As one of the nightshade family of plants, however, peppers are perhaps best avoided by those with joint problems.

· · · · · · · · · · · · · · · · ·

Recommended for:
cancer
circulatory
respiratory
skin

Tomatoes

★ ★ ★ ★

All of the tomatoes we eat today are descendants of the cherry tomatoes that have always grown wild along the western coast of South America. The Mexicans were probably the first to cultivate the tomato, and from Mexico, this fleshy fruit was introduced to Europe by the Spanish during the 16th century. After this, the tomato rapidly became popular across the south of Europe. Since they are members of the deadly nightshade family, tomatoes were treated with suspicion at first, but they soon became an integral component of cuisines all around the Mediterranean.

Tomatoes are very rich in antioxidants, especially beta-carotene and lycopene, and they also contain a good deal of vitamins C and E. This makes them good for the cardiovascular system. Research shows that they may also help to prevent some forms of cancer, particularly prostate cancer. Lycopene seems to protect men against this form of cancer, which is far less common in Mediterranean countries, where men may eat as many as 6–8 ripe tomatoes a day. Fortunately, in this age of processed food, processed tomatoes actually contain far more lycopene than fresh ones, so tinned tomatoes, tomato sauce, sun-dried tomatoes, and even ketchup are important sources of this antioxidant. Tomatoes are also low in sodium and rich in potassium, making them good for conditions such as high blood pressure and fluid retention.

In the largest study to date, it was evident that eating four portions of tomato sauce weekly reduced prostate cancer risk by 35 per cent. Although lycopene may be useful as a supplement, research shows that when tomato products are cooked and combined with oil, the lycopene is more biologically available – so pills aren't a substitute for the real thing. There are other plant chemicals in tomatoes that are also cancer-protective.

A ripe tomato contains more than 200 volatile compounds that make up its unique taste and smell. Green tomatoes contain a chemical called tomatine, which may trigger migraine attacks if you're a sufferer. Tomatine is destroyed by cooking but remains in quite high amounts in the pickled green tomatoes popular in the US.

There should always be a few tins of tomatoes in your cupboard, as they lose very little of their nutritional value during tinning and are a great standby for instant high-nutrient sauces.

• • • • • • • • • • • • • • • • • • • •

Recommended for:
cancer
respiratory
skin

Pumpkin and squash

★★★★

Pumpkin and squash were an important part of the diet of many Native American tribes, who introduced them to the early European settlers. In North America, squash and pumpkin (especially in the form of pumpkin pie) are still served as part of the traditional Thanksgiving meal. These vegetables are not only delicious, but are also filling, inexpensive, high-energy foods.

As you might expect from their wonderful deep orange hue, pumpkins and squashes are full of beta-carotene, the vitamin A precursor that helps protect us against cancer, heart troubles, and respiratory disease. In population studies, people eating plenty of pumpkin, or other orange-yellow members of the squash family, run a lower risk of developing lung cancer.

• • • • • • • • • • • • • • • • • • • •

Recommended for:
cancer
circulatory
respiratory
skin

Carrots

Carrots are so rich in beta-carotene that a single "old" carrot supplies enough vitamin A for an entire day. Carrots are also near the top of the list of vegetables that protect us against cancer, and especially against lung cancer, a fact that is borne out in a number of population studies.

In traditional country wisdom favoured by many orthodox French physicians, a purée of cooked carrots is the perfect answer to infant diarrhoea, suggesting that carrots have an antibiotic as well as a nutritive action.

A two- or three-day fast, taking nothing but water and raw carrot juice, has been recommended for liver problems, and carrot juice is equally valuable for jaundice. Eating carrots increases the levels of red blood cells, and studies have also shown that carrots protect against excess ultraviolet light or radiation. Their antioxidant content is also useful for people with atherosclerosis (narrowed arteries).

Recommended for:
cancer
circulatory
digestive
respiratory

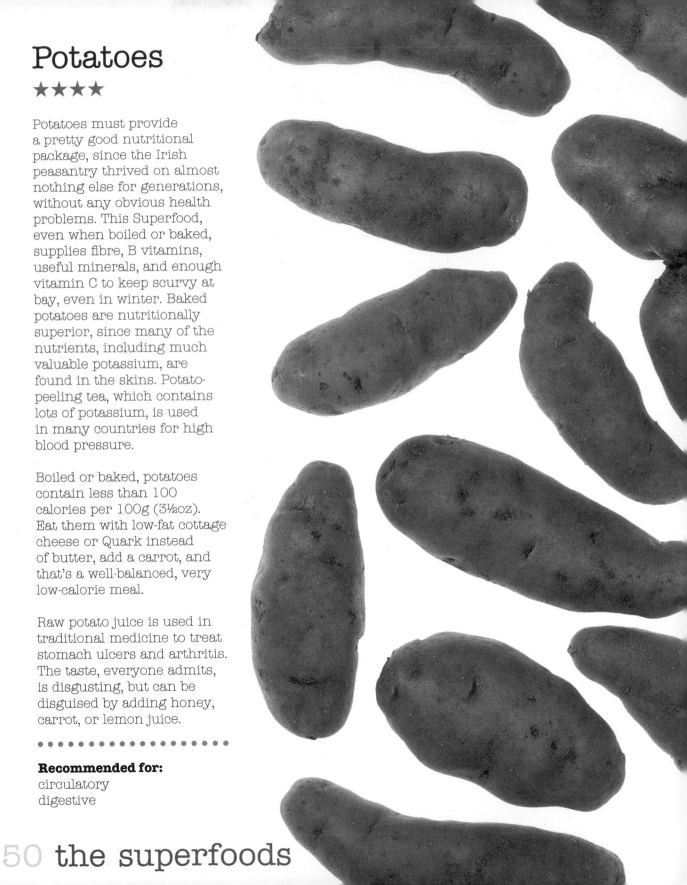

Potatoes
★★★★

Potatoes must provide
a pretty good nutritional
package, since the Irish
peasantry thrived on almost
nothing else for generations,
without any obvious health
problems. This Superfood,
even when boiled or baked,
supplies fibre, B vitamins,
useful minerals, and enough
vitamin C to keep scurvy at
bay, even in winter. Baked
potatoes are nutritionally
superior, since many of the
nutrients, including much
valuable potassium, are
found in the skins. Potato-
peeling tea, which contains
lots of potassium, is used
in many countries for high
blood pressure.

Boiled or baked, potatoes
contain less than 100
calories per 100g (3½oz).
Eat them with low-fat cottage
cheese or Quark instead
of butter, add a carrot, and
that's a well-balanced, very
low-calorie meal.

Raw potato juice is used in
traditional medicine to treat
stomach ulcers and arthritis.
The taste, everyone admits,
is disgusting, but can be
disguised by adding honey,
carrot, or lemon juice.

. . . .

Recommended for:
circulatory
digestive

Sweet potatoes

★★★★

Sweet potatoes are an excellent source of energy, providing some protein, vitamin C and E, and lots of carotenoids, including beta-carotene. They are a powerful anti-cancer food, with one serving a day reducing the risk of lung cancer. This is even more important if you are a smoker or an ex-smoker.

Sweet potatoes are an extremely versatile vegetable and are wonderfully healthy for children and adults alike. A good way to introduce them to your family is to peel and cube a sweet potato and cook it together with ordinary potatoes, drain them, and mash with a little butter or olive oil and some grated nutmeg. They're equally delicious mashed together with parsnip or swede. They're also great roasted in a medium oven brushed with olive oil and a little black pepper. One of our favourite juices is apple, carrot, celery, and sweet potato, which tastes better than it sounds.

● ● ● ● ● ● ● ● ● ● ● ● ● ● ● ● ●

Recommended for:
cancer
digestive
fatigue
respiratory

Swedes

★★★★

Another of the large and health-giving crucifer family, swede is often thought of as no more than cattle fodder. However, it's an excellent vegetable with a delicate flavour and all the anti-cancer properties of this family of plants. It contains protective phytochemicals and significant amounts of vitamin C, with a serving providing 75 per cent of the UK RDA, useful amounts of vitamin A, almost no sodium, a little fibre, and small amounts of trace minerals. Swede supplies only 24 calories per serving, but lots of satisfying bulk, making it a real bonus for those watching their weight.

Mashed together with potato, swedes produce a most interesting and flavoursome variation on the usual dish and are an excellent early weaning food for babies.

Note that, like other cruciferae, swedes contain goiterogens and should be eaten in moderation by anyone with thyroid problems or taking long-term thyroxin treatment.

• • • • • • • • • • • • • • • • • •

Recommended for:
cancer
skin

Turnips

★★★★

Turnips are one of the oldest of all the cultivated vegetables, and have been a staple of the peasant diet in cold, northern European countries for many centuries. They supply plenty of energy-giving carbohydrate, along with reasonable amounts of many nutrients, including vitamins C and B6. The tops or greens are as healthy as the turnips themselves, and are best when eaten young and fresh.

Turnips are warmly recommended for gout in traditional medicine, as they are eliminators of uric acid. A thin purée of turnips, cooked in milk, is an old country remedy for bronchitis: the sulphurous compound raphanol may be responsible for this bactericidal action. It would be surprising, too, if a member of the powerful crucifer family were devoid of such healing and antibiotic powers.

Recommended for:
joints
respiratory

53

Beetroot

★★★★

In Romany medicine, beetroot juice was used as a blood-builder for patients who were pale and run-down, and in Russia and Eastern Europe it's used both to build up resistance and to treat convalescents after a serious illness. In the traditional medicine of Central Europe, beetroot has a long history of use in the treatment of cancer: it seems to contain anti-carcinogens bound to the red colouring matter, as well as possessing a striking ability to increase cellular uptake of oxygen. Many of these actions are enhanced when the beetroot is eaten raw or drunk as juice. The popular French starter crudités – which combine grated raw beetroot, raw carrot, and perhaps paper-thin slices of cucumber, all dressed with olive oil and lemon juice and garnished with chopped parsley – is a more powerful tonic for general health than a whole bottle of vitamin pills.

• • • • • • • • • • • • • • • •

Recommended for:
cancer
digestive
fatigue

Parsnips

★★★★

The wild parsnip has been used for centuries in Europe, where it grows around the borders of cultivated fields and in chalky soil in roadside verges. Like carrots, parsnips have long been a popular cultivated vegetable with a history of countryside use. In Germany they're often eaten with salted fish during Lent; in Holland they're used for soup; in Ireland they were boiled with water and hops for beer; and in England countrywomen made them into jam and parsnip wine.

The great herbalists, such as Culpeper, were all fans of the humble parsnip and advised giving it to humans as well as livestock. Parsnips provide calories, fibre, potassium, folic acid, vitamin E, and traces of minerals and other B vitamins. They taste best after the first hard frosts of winter. Mash them together with swede, carrot, or potato, or brush them with a little oil and roast. They're even fabulous cooked on the barbecue.

• • • • • • • • • • • • • • • •

Recommended for:
circulatory
digestive
fatigue

Jerusalem artichokes

★★★★

Jerusalem artichokes belong to the sunflower family and Italians call them "girasole". "Jerusalem" appears to be a corruption of the Italian word. By the 1800s they were popular in England made into "Palestine Soup".

Rich in carbohydrates, there is little sugar in them as they contain inulin, which the body deals with in the same way as fibre. Inulin isn't broken down during normal digestion but ends up in the large bowel (colon), where it provides food for billions of friendly probiotic bacteria. As with globe artichokes, the resulting fermentation can sometimes be a cause of wind, but that's a small price to pay for the fabulous taste and the low glycaemic index benefits of this much underrated vegetable. Jerusalem artichokes are ideal for diabetics and anyone who has problems keeping their blood sugar levels on an even keel, as they are filling and satisfying, and the inulin is not absorbed by the body.

Jerusalem artichokes are extremely low in calories – only 78 per 100g (3½oz) – and contain hardly any salt but are a rich source of heart-friendly potassium. They also provide useful quantities of iron and some B vitamins. Dried and ground into flour, they are perfect for anyone with gluten, wheat, or other cereal allergies.

Recommended for:
circulatory
digestion
fatigue

Globe artichokes

★★★★

Globe artichokes, as any Frenchman will tell you, are the friend of the liver. In 1975 three Frenchwomen, specialists in pharmacy, published a study of plants used in modern medicine; they listed no less than 51 different pharmaceutical preparations based on the leaves of this plant. The active compound that seems to be chiefly responsible is called cynarine, which acts powerfully on the liver to promote the flow of bile and stimulate liver cell regeneration.

These healing powers are concentrated mainly in the leaf, and when you buy artichokes in a continental market, they are sold complete with stem and leaves for those who wish to avail themselves of this excellent natural medicine. The globes, too, share some of this curative potential, making artichokes a Superfood for anyone with liver or digestive problems.

The artichoke is also a friend to the heart. In European folk medicine, it's used to treat high blood pressure and ward off heart attacks; studies have shown that artichokes have a distinct cholesterol-lowering ability, as well as a marked diuretic effect.

All of these qualities make artichokes one of the great purifying and detoxifying plants, particularly useful for those with rheumatism, arthritis, or gout.

Recommended for:
circulatory
digestive
joints

Onions

★★★★

Onions belong to the same botanical family as garlic, and both are the subject of intensive modern medical research, which only confirms the high reputation as a cure-all that they have always enjoyed. With garlic, onions share a protective action on the circulatory system that is fascinating cardiologists the world over. In a delightful trial carried out at Newcastle's Royal Victoria Infirmary, 22 volunteers were first asked to fast and then fed fried fatty British breakfasts, starring bacon and eggs. Half the volunteers had a little extra something on the menu: a helping of fried onions. When post-breakfast blood samples from both lots of breakfasters were analysed, they showed a startling difference. In people who ate the fry-up feasts without onions, the blood samples showed an increasing tendency to clot – a state which could eventually lead to life-threatening thrombosis. The blood of the onion-eaters, however – despite all that bacon and egg – showed a reduced tendency to clot. In a similar study in India, rich, fatty food pushed up blood cholesterol levels, and onions, whether cooked or raw, pulled it right back down. Dr Victor Gurewitch of Tufts University in the US has found that eating just half an onion daily – raw, please, not cooked – can raise blood levels of beneficial high-density lipoproteins by an average of 30 per cent.

Onions are impressive country medicine for a huge range of ailments – among them anaemia, arthritis and rheumatism, gout, and premature aging. They star in hundreds of traditional recipes, like this one for colic in babies: slice an onion, infuse it in hot water for a few minutes, let it cool, and give the baby a teaspoonful of the water. And onion soup at the end of a night on the tiles is part of Paris mythology.

Many of the onion's traditional properties are now being confirmed by modern research. In studies with rabbits, subcutaneous injections of onion extract lowered blood sugar levels more slowly than insulin, but for a longer period. It is thought this action is due to the glucokinine in onions. In other trials, onions were found to be effective against asthma. They are strongly diuretic, dissolving and eliminating urea, and they have powerful antibiotic activity.

• •

Recommended for:
circulatory
digestive
fatigue
respiratory
urinary

Leeks

★★★★

Leeks have been cultivated in the West for at least 4000 years, and the ancient Egyptians, the ancient Greeks, and the Romans all prized them for their medicinal value. Members of the same healing family as onions and garlic, they have the same therapeutic properties, although in a milder form. In French traditional medicine they are prescribed for respiratory problems, and being rich in potassium, they are also valued for their cleansing, diuretic powers. Their ability to eliminate uric acid means that people with gout or arthritis should eat plenty of leeks.

• • • • • • • • • • • • • • • • • •

Recommended for:
joints
respiratory
urinary

Spinach

This vegetable is iron-rich, as every admirer of Popeye knows. Orthodox nutritionists, however, point out crushingly that the iron in cooked spinach is poorly absorbed by the body. This is because spinach has high levels of oxalic acid, which interact with magnesium and calcium to carry it out of the body in the form of insoluble salts. Spinach is also rich in uric acid, so it is best avoided by the gouty and the rheumatic.

Spinach is very rich in the dark green plant "blood" chlorophyll (*Red cabbage, p.62*), so anaemia patients or those suffering from fatigue and mental strain should eat plenty of it, raw, in the form of salads.

Cancer patients, or those at risk from cancer such as heavy smokers, should include plenty of raw spinach in their diets, too. Cancer research is increasingly focusing on the whole spectrum of carotenoids – not just beta-carotene – in dark green or brightly coloured fruits and vegetables, and spinach is more highly endowed with those potential cancer-fighters than even carrots. In population studies quoted by Jean Carper, dark green vegetables, with spinach at the top of the list, are strongly protective against cancer.

Recommended for:
cancer
stress
fatigue

Red cabbage

★★★★

Cabbage has been the subject of an impressive amount of medical research. This is not surprising: its healing powers, which are long attested in traditional medicine, cover an amazing range of ailments.

Cabbage contains healing mucilaginous substances similar to those produced by the mucous membrane of the gut and stomach for their own protection. This confirms the effectiveness of the traditional raw cabbage-juice cure for ulcers. Cabbage is also loaded with sulphur compounds that, according to Dr Valnet, give it a tonic and disinfectant action in respiratory infections.

Anyone who is anaemic should eat cabbage for its iron and chlorophyll, the green "blood" of plants, which is chemically similar to the haemoglobin in human blood. Leslie Kenton quotes studies in which the red blood cells of anaemic rabbits were restored to normal after being fed crude chlorophyll for a fortnight. Centuries of use have also given the cabbage a reputation as being protective against stress, infection, and cardiac problems, while as a member of the crucifer family, it is known to contain many anti-cancer compounds. In population studies, people eating the most cabbage were the least likely to develop cancers. Perhaps even more excitingly, 50 per cent of guinea pigs fed diced raw cabbage before whole body irradiation survived, while those that were not so protected all died within 15 days. So maybe all those working with VDU screens, or facing radiation treatment or even diagnostic X-rays, should eat plenty of raw cabbage.

Most of these therapeutic effects have been observed with raw cabbage, and no doubt would also be found in sauerkraut. Traditional boiling in water not only means major nutrient losses into the water, but the disappearance or deactivation of many healing compounds. Cooked cabbage is rough on the digestion, too. So cook cabbage in its own juices, for as short a time as possible.

Recommended for:
cancer
circulatory
digestive
respiratory

63

Sauerkraut

In traditional European sauerkraut, raw cabbage is finely shredded and layered in a stone crock, with sea salt and spices. By the time the crock is full, the cabbage juices have fermented to produce a sour taste.

All over Europe, sauerkraut has been a dietary staple of the peasantry: a good way of preserving the autumn cabbages so that they could be eaten through the winter. Sauerkraut can truly be called a wonderfood: since the enzymes and vitamin C of cabbage are well preserved in it, it must have saved millions from scurvy.

Apart from being high in vitamin C, sauerkraut is also rich in calcium and a good source of potassium. Sauerkraut is traditionally a medicine too, in both preventative and curative senses. Dyspepsia, arthritis, cold, indigestion, stomach ulcers, skin problems – all were treated with sauerkraut and it was often very effective. We now know why.

Any toxins brewing in our gut may prepare the ground for a number of serious diseases. Not for sauerkraut-eaters, though, since the lactic acid that forms during fermentation does a wonderful clean-up job in the digestive tract. Benevolent bacteria multiply, killing off excess bad bacteria to produce a healthy colon once more.

• •

Recommended for:
cancer
digestive
joints

Oriental greens

★★★★

The Oriental leaves, such as pak choi, make a tasty, nutritious, and interesting contribution to healthy eating. They are superfoods in every sense, as they're extremely easy to grow, with many of them being suitable as a cut-and-come-again plant in the garden or greenhouse. Raw, stir-fried, steamed, braised, in salads, or in combination recipes, they're extremely versatile. Dark leaves contain the most beta-carotene, which is converted into vitamin A – important for the skin, immune health, and eyesight.

As members of the carotenoid family, Oriental greens protect against some cancers, particularly lung cancer. They also help to maintain vision and protect against age-related macular degeneration, which is the most common cause of visual deterioration in elderly people. These green leaves also provide valuable amounts of vitamin C, with one-third of the daily requirement delivered in an average portion, as well as some folic acid.

One of the most popular of the Oriental greens is Chinese cabbage, which is best served raw, lightly steamed, or stir-fried. Boiling it is a crime! Mizuna, with its peppery taste, is used raw, stir-fried, or in soup, and pak choi, widely available, can be eaten raw when young.

• •

Recommended for:
skin
cancer

Asparagus

★★★★

Asparagus has somehow become infamous for the strange odour produced by your urine after you eat it: this area has not been tremendously well researched. In 1891 a scientist called Nencki asserted that the smell was due to a metabolite called methanethiol, and although other theories have arisen since, none seems to have won the day so far.

Asparagus really benefits the kidneys and the liver, and as it promotes elimination through the urine, it is warmly recommended for people who have rheumatism and arthritis. It's also a great source of folate, a B vitamin that is good for your cardiovascular system and is especially important for pregnant women, because it's known to help prevent certain birth defects, such as spina bifida. You can save the water asparagus is cooked in and drink it as a useful diuretic. Since asparagus is high in purines, people who suffer from gout should avoid it.

Recommended for:
digestive
joints
urinary

Broccoli

★★★★

Broccoli is a cruciferous plant with cancer-protective properties. Six major population studies analyzed at the US National Cancer Institute showed that the more cruciferous vegetables (including cauliflower, radishes, horseradish, cabbage, spring greens, turnips, Brussels sprouts, and kale) you eat, the lower your chances of developing bowel cancer – a finding now reinforced by the American Institute of Cancer Research.

Broccoli is an excellent source of fibre, folate, and vitamins A and C. It's a very good source of potassium, B2, and B6 and contains reasonable amounts of iron, calcium, and vitamin E. Cruciferous vegetables also suppress free-radical formation, making them good for joints and the heart.

Recent studies reveal that broccoli helps to destroy damaged cells, helps prostate cancer, prevents cataracts, and builds stronger bones.

• • • • • • • • • • • • • • • • • •

Recommended for:
cancer
circulatory
joints

Barley

★★★★

Barley has been cultivated longer than any other cereal. Bread made from barley was a staple in the Middle Ages, but was so heavy that it fell out of favour and was superseded first by oats and then by wheat. Barley has always been highly valued for its uniquely soothing qualities when used to treat inflammatory conditions of the intestines and urinary tract. Herbalists recommend plenty of barley water to help counter the painful irritation of cystitis and constipation.

Like other grains, barley is mineral-rich, with particularly high levels of calcium and potassium, and plenty of B-complex vitamins. This makes it useful for people suffering from stress or fatigue and a nourishing food for convalescence. Research on the cholesterol-lowering effect of cereals – wheat, rye, oats, and barley – have found that their coarse outer layers are rich in substances that inhibit the synthesis of cholesterol by the liver.

Nutritionally, however, pot barley – the little, beige, dehulled grains – is highly superior to cleaned or pearl barley. Use barley in soups, as stuffing for poultry, or eat it cooked on its own. You can also use it to make a delicious bread.

• •

Recommended for:
circulatory
digestive
stress
fatigue
urinary

Brown rice

★★★★

Rice is a marvellous complete food, the dietary staple of the East. Until the advent of rice-milling, it was eaten unpolished. With the new, milled white rice came a disastrous epidemic of beriberi – a disease of the brain and nervous system – that spread like wildfire around the Eastern world. Beriberi is caused by deficiency of a B vitamin, thiamine, in which the rice-polishings are rich, so white rice today is sometimes "parboiled" or "converted" by a process of steaming to drive some of the vitamins back into the grain.

Plain boiled brown rice is a universal folk remedy for diarrhoea, as is the water in which rice is boiled, which is also recommended for fevers. It seems to have a beneficial effect on the entire intestinal tract, soothing and cleansing it. A regime of plain, boiled, unsalted rice is warmly recommended by French doctors for lowering the blood pressure. To this can be added a purée of apples.

Rice should be washed in running water before cooking, but never soaked, since vital minerals and vitamins leach out with the dirt.

Recommended for:
circulatory
digestive
stress
fatigue

Buckwheat

★★★★

Buckwheat, often considered a grain, is actually a seed related to rhubarb. In Russia and Poland it is a diet staple. Considering the harsh climate in these countries, this makes a lot of sense. Buckwheat is high in a flavonoid called glycoside rutin, which strengthens and tones the walls of the capillaries, the tiniest blood vessels in your body, and so protects against frostbite and chilblains. Buckwheat helps high blood pressure and atherosclerosis. Protein-rich and gluten-free, it's excellent for people with coeliac disease.

Recommended for:
circulatory
digestive
stress

Lentils

★★★★

This pulse is rich in protein, minerals, and fibre, is a good source of B vitamins, and is very low in fat. These complex carbohydrates are now recommended to us by cardiologists and slimming specialists alike. Lentils are a diet staple the world over, often served with grains such as barley. This pairing maximizes protein consumption, since together, they contain a better balance of the eight amino acids. Flavour lentils with herbs and spices such as cumin, fennel, and garlic, which help to counter flatulence.

Recommended for:
circulatory
fatigue

Beans

Dried beans (pulses) are the second largest group of foods forming man's diet. Weight for weight they contain almost as much protein as fillet steak, at a fraction of the cost and with many more health benefits.

Beans help to reduce cholesterol and protect against heart disease, circulatory problems, and bowel cancer. With a low GI, they provide slow-release energy, making them excellent for diabetics. They are also rich in plant hormones (phytoestrogens), which protect against osteoporosis and breast and prostate cancers.

Soybeans (*p. 71*) are the best vegetable source of protein, with the highest phytoestrogen content and the strongest antioxidant activity. This protects against both heart disease and cancer.

Other beans have individual properties (*see below*) and a variety of flavours that make them all valuable.

Pinto potassium, fibre, folate.
Mung less starch, more folate.
Kidney fibre, potassium, zinc.
Haricot fibre, iron.
Chickpeas fibre, calcium, iron, zinc.
Butter fibre, potassium, iron.
Blackeyed fibre, selenium, folate.
Baked beans fibre, iron, selenium, iodine – but beware the salt.
Aduki fibre, magnesium, potassium, zinc.

Recommended for:
cancer
circulatory
fatigue

Millet

★★★★

Millet is the only grain that is a complete protein. It is also the only alkaline grain, making it particularly suitable for invalids and growing children.

It is also rich in silicon, a structural part of collagen (the tough substance that holds us together). Silicon is vital for the health of hair, skin, teeth, eyes, and nails. A lack of it can result in sagging connective tissue. Clogged arteries have much lower levels of silicon than disease-free arteries, so it seems to benefit arterial health.

• •

Recommended for:
circulatory
fatigue
skin

Maize

★★★★

Maize grows all over the world and is the staple food of millions. It is gluten-free and is used for many products – cornflakes, popcorn, cornflour, polenta, grits, and tortillas, which are all suitable for coeliacs.

Diets dependent on maize, however, can cause the deficiency disease pellagra, in which the body gets too little of the B vitamin nicotinic acid. Maize is deficient in tryptophan, which is essential for the absorption of this B vitamin.

• •

Recommended for:
digestive

Oats

★★★★

Oats contain a lot of protein for a grain. They also contain polyunsaturated fats, vitamin E, and B vitamins. They are very high in calcium, potassium, and magnesium, which, like the B vitamins, are vital to a healthy nervous system, as well as to strong bones and teeth. Oats also supply silicon for healthy arterial walls. They also protect the digestive surfaces and soothe the stomach and intestines.

Oats have an impressive reputation in traditional medicine. Possets and caudles made from oatmeal with water, lemon juice, sugar, spices, and perhaps ale or wine, were for centuries a prescription for any sickroom, along with gruel or porridge.

Herbalists turn to oats for one of their most reliable remedies for depression and general debility – a tincture of the whole plant, or just the dehusked oat. So potent is its tranquillizing effect that it is now being used by a number of health practitioners to wean people off the man-made tranquillizers to which so many thousands are addicted.

In dozens of studies, the cholesterol levels of patients fed a daily dose of oat-bran have declined an average 20 per cent. The glutinous fibre in the oat-bran appears to remove bile acids that would otherwise be converted into cholesterol. Oats should certainly figure on the diabetic's menu too, since they appear to have a very favourable effect on the metabolism of sugar.

• •

Recommended for:
circulatory
digestive
fatigue
stress

Soybeans

★★★★

Soybeans are extraordinarily high in protein, well-absorbed iron and calcium, B vitamins, and lecithin (a natural emulsifier of fats that lowers cholesterol). Soybeans turn up in a number of different disguises: as flour; as a milk substitute; sprouted; or fermented to produce miso, shoyu, and tofu. They also turn up disguised as meat and are used as a substitute in pies, sausages, and casseroles. In our view, this is a long way from what either healthy eating or the enjoyment of food is about.

It may not be as healthy to rely heavily on soy, as many people suggest: reports suggest that they contain a thyroid-depressing element. Annemarie Colbin points out that the Japanese eat tofu in only small amounts, with rice as their staple, and that they eat iodine-rich seaweed almost daily, by way of instinctive compensation. Eat soybeans in moderation, therefore, if you want to benefit from their very real nutritional bonuses.

Recommended for:
cancer
circulation
stress

Wheat
★ ★ ★ ★

When most people say bread, they mean bread made from wheat flour, which is rich in zinc, magnesium, vitamin B6, pyridoxine, vitamin E, and fibre. But there is bread and there is bread. It is a long way from the loaf baked from the freshly milled wholegrain of organically grown wheat, with no additions other than salt and yeast, to the flabby white stuff made with any number of additives, from wheat produced by agrofarming, in which pesticide residues may linger, and which has had much of its goodness refined out of it.

Frumenty, made from wheat grains, is one of the most ancient of English dishes. Sprouted wheat, which is nutritionally even richer, is recommended for cancer patients.

A number of people are wheat-intolerant. For many of them, the problem lies not in the wheat itself but in pesticide residues found in it. They should experiment with bread from organically grown wheat.

Recommended for:
circulatory
stress

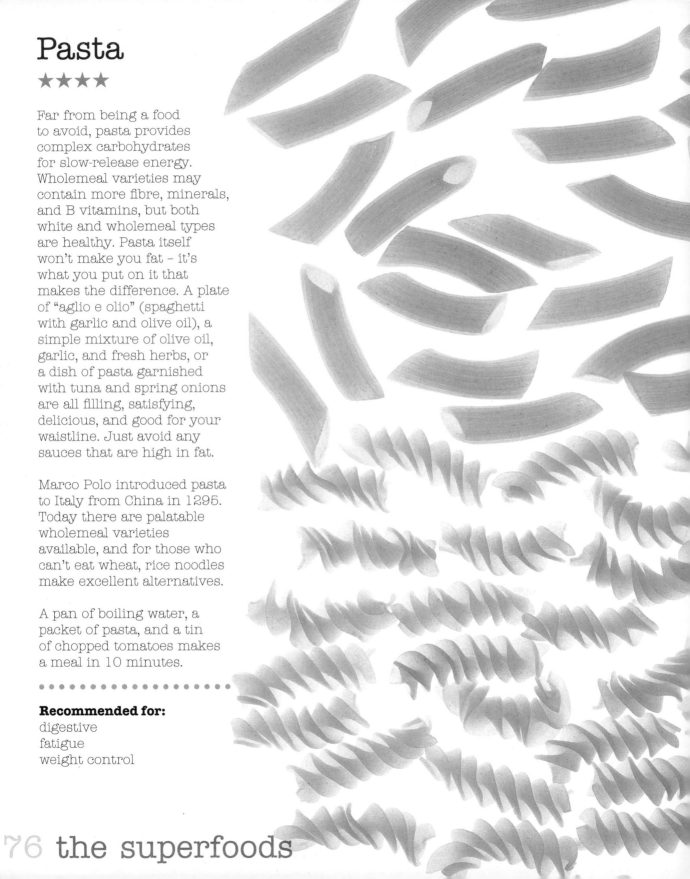

Pasta

★★★★

Far from being a food to avoid, pasta provides complex carbohydrates for slow-release energy. Wholemeal varieties may contain more fibre, minerals, and B vitamins, but both white and wholemeal types are healthy. Pasta itself won't make you fat – it's what you put on it that makes the difference. A plate of "aglio e olio" (spaghetti with garlic and olive oil), a simple mixture of olive oil, garlic, and fresh herbs, or a dish of pasta garnished with tuna and spring onions are all filling, satisfying, delicious, and good for your waistline. Just avoid any sauces that are high in fat.

Marco Polo introduced pasta to Italy from China in 1295. Today there are palatable wholemeal varieties available, and for those who can't eat wheat, rice noodles make excellent alternatives.

A pan of boiling water, a packet of pasta, and a tin of chopped tomatoes makes a meal in 10 minutes.

• • • • • • • • • • • • • • • • • • •

Recommended for:
digestive
fatigue
weight control

Bread

★★★★

Good bread is indeed "the staff of life" and an important part of a healthy, balanced diet. Wholemeal bread contains five times as much fibre as white bread, and valuable amounts of vitamin E, potassium, iron, zinc, copper, magnesium, thiamin, riboflavin, pantothenic acid, folic acid, pyridoxine, and biotin. You'll also get 10 times as much manganese, twice as much chromium, and one and a half times as much selenium as you will from white bread.

The best way to avoid the high salt content in commercial bread is by making your own. It's one of the most satisfying things you can ever do in a kitchen. But if you can't be bothered with proving, kneading, and pummelling, you could buy a bread machine instead. Either way, you'll be able to control what goes into your daily bread.

● ● ● ● ● ● ● ● ● ● ● ● ● ● ● ● ●

Recommended for:
digestive
stress
fatigue

Almonds

★★★★

Almonds are not really nuts as we always imagine; they are, in fact, the seed of the fruit of the almond tree. Most importantly, almonds are a highly concentrated food that is rich in protein, fat, and vital minerals such as zinc, magnesium, potassium, and iron, as well as some B vitamins. Since they are also high in oxalic and phytic acid, which combine with these minerals to carry them out of your body, you should eat them at the same time as vitamin-C rich foods for maximum absorption.

Almonds are 20 per cent protein – weight for weight, they have one-third more protein than eggs. The oil in almonds is soothing, and almond milk is a classic sickroom drink, being both sustaining and soothing. It is recommended by herbalists for respiratory ailments as well as digestive upsets. Almond milk can be combined with barley water for urinary problems. Dr Valnet has a recipe for making almond milk: soak 60g (2oz) whole almonds in tepid water, then skin them. Measure out 900ml (1½pt) of water, and pound the almonds with a few tablespoons of the water (you can do this easily in a food processor), adding the rest of the water once you've produced a paste. Add a tablespoon of honey, and strain through muslin.

Recommended for:
digestive
respiratory
urinary

Cashews

This delicious nut is always sold shelled. Avoid the salted ones and choose the plain roasted variety instead. Cashews, like olive oil, are high in healthy heart-protecting monounsaturated fats. Whizzed in a processor with a little walnut oil, they make wonderful cashew nut butter. They're also a very good source of copper and a good source of magnesium, tryptophan, and protein. Cashews also contain some folic acid, potassium, and fibre.

Rcommcndod for:
circulatory
digestive
stress
fatigue

Hazelnuts

Deliciously crunchy hazelnuts can be bought ready-shelled to eat as a nourishing snack. They contain the B vitamin thiamine (deficiency of which can make you feel low and lethargic) and they also supply the omega-3 fats needed to balance omega-6 fats in our diets. Dry roast hazelnuts in a hot frying pan, chop them, and sprinkle on fruit or green salads. They're a good source of protein and also contain fibre, magnesium, and vitamin E.

Recommended for:
fatigue
stress
joints

Pumpkin seeds

★★★★

Pumpkin seeds contain measurable amounts of zinc, iron, and calcium, and they're an excellent snack food, supplying protein and B-complex vitamins. In traditional medicine in many parts of the world, particularly in Eastern Europe, they also have a high reputation as a male sexual tonic and protector of the prostate gland.

For prostate disorders, Russians simmer 100g (3½oz) of the unshelled seeds in 750ml (1¼pt) of water for 20 minutes and take a wineglassful three times a day. The protective action of pumpkin seeds has been ascribed to a plant hormone that is found in them, but more research in this area is needed.

Recommended for:
stress
fatigue
skin

Sesame seeds

★★★★

These little seeds are the vegetarian's friend. A large handful will supply about 26 grams of protein, or about two-thirds of a day's needs for a reasonably active man. Unusually for vegetable sources, they are also rich in the amino acids methionine and tryptophan, which are important for good liver and kidney health. They are also well endowed with minerals, containing over 7mg iron and 10.3mg zinc per 100g (3½oz). Eat a vitamin C-rich fruit or vegetable at the same meal, though, to help your body absorb the minerals. Sesame seeds are also a good source of polyunsaturated fatty acids and vitamin E.

In ancient Babylon – as today all over the Arab world – halvah was made from pounded sesame seeds and honey and eaten to enhance sexual vitality. Paavo Airla, one of the US's most highly respected naturopaths, listed sesame seeds among ten foods for maintaining and enhancing sexual vigour.

• • • • • • • • • • • • • • • • •

Recommended for:
circulatory
fatigue

Sprouted seeds

★★★★

Sprouted seeds are a wonderful source of vitamins and minerals. They have been described as "the most live, pure, nutritious food imaginable". They are cheap and easy to grow even if you don't own so much as a window box, and if you sprout them yourself, you can be sure that they are organic, produced without fertilizers or pesticides.

When you sprout beans or seeds, what you produce is an enormously enhanced package of the nutrients already present in the original seeds. This can include the full range of vitamins and minerals, plus a powerhouse of plant enzymes, which are at their most abundant in the early sprouting stage. Plant enzymes are thought to activate the body's own enzyme systems and boost the ability to metabolize fats and oils.

One researcher found that levels of vitamin B2 in oats rose by 1300 per cent almost as soon as they began sprouting, and by the time green leaves formed, the increase was 2000 per cent. B6 (pyridoxine) was up 500 per cent, and folic acid 600 per cent. In one study, only small amounts of vitamin C were found in unsprouted wheat grains, and this increased by 600 per cent while sprouting over the next few days.

Their wealth of 100 per cent natural nutrition, free of chemical pollution, makes sprouts an obvious choice for cancer patients. They are used extensively at many clinics practising the natural approach to treating cancer. They are also valuable for anyone anxious to boost their immune defences, and for all conditions needing first-class nutrition.

More and more supermarkets are now selling sprouted seeds. If your local one doesn't, or only stocks one or two kinds, write to the manager suggesting that they extend their range.

• •

Recommended for:
cancer
stress
fatigue
skin

the superfoods

Sunflower seeds

★★★★

These seeds are concentrated nourishment, containing protein, B-complex vitamins, and useful levels of minerals. They are also rich in polyunsaturated oils, which is why you should examine hulled nuts carefully before you eat them: they easily turn rancid, when they become a most unhealthy food. Fresh hulled nuts are a pale, uniform grey – rancid ones are yellow brown. Buy unshelled sunflower seeds, and enjoy cracking them open to find the fresh nuts the way children do all around the Mediterranean.

Eaten regularly, sunflower seeds will help to counter fatigue, depression, irritability, and lack of energy. Smokers trying to give up the habit find chewing them particularly helpful. They're also an excellent addition to the school lunchbox.

Recommended for:
stress
fatigue

Walnuts

★★★★

Walnuts are protein-rich, containing as much protein, weight for weight, as eggs. They are also high in potassium and other minerals, such as zinc and iron. Eat them in salads, where vitamin C-rich foods will help your body absorb these minerals.

Recommended for:
circulatory
fatigue

Chestnuts

Chestnuts must be cooked and can then be added to sweet and savoury dishes, soups, stuffings, or vegetables. Try them with Brussels sprouts or broccoli and Stilton soup. Unlike other nuts, they contain virtually no fat and only 170 calories per 100g (3½oz). Because they're high in starch, they can be dried and ground into excellent gluten-free flour. They don't supply much protein, but they do contain the B vitamins thiamin (B1), riboflavin (B2), and pyridoxine (B6), and potassium.

Recommended for:
circulatory
fatigue

Peanuts

A large-scale experiment has shown that a teaspoon of peanut butter five days a week produces an average pound a week weight loss. The monounsaturated fats reduce cholesterol and prevent heart disease. With a very low glycaemic index rating, peanuts may also help to prevent adult-onset diabetes, as they hardly raise blood-sugar levels. They also provide vitamin B3, folate, and protein. Peanuts and organic peanut butter should be part of a healthy diet.

Recommended for:
circulatory
fatigue

Milk

★★★★

Cow's milk is extremely nutritious, a first-class protein, and a rich source of calcium. It also provides some B vitamins and a little iron and zinc. As a fast food, and as a regular part of a child's diet, it can be warmly recommended.

Milk, however, is a fatty food. If you order skimmed milk to avoid the fat, you also lose the vitamins A, D, and E present in whole milk. Moreover, the mineral calcium needs to be in balance with another important mineral, magnesium, deficiency of which is very common in modern Western diets; and milk is a poor source of magnesium.

A number of adults – and whole populations in the eastern and southern hemispheres – lack the digestive enzyme lactase, which is needed in order to absorb all the goodies in milk. Many more people may be intolerant to milk, and to other dairy products such as butter and cheese. So milk is not a Superfood for everyone.

• • • • • • • • • • • • • • • • • •

Recommended for:
stress
joints

Yoghurt

★★★★

Yoghurt is a valuable food for your digestive system. When the natural balance between beneficial and harmful bacteria in the gut is upset, it can lead to fermentation, wind, putrefaction, constipation, and poor absorption. If ignored, this may give rise to even more severe health problems. Live yoghurt contains *Lactobacillus bulgaricus*, a microbe which helps restore equilibrium in the gut.

Yoghurt's lactic acids aid digestion by synthesizing B vitamins and increasing the uptake of nutrients, particularly of calcium (which yoghurt also supplies). They regulate bowel function, and have properties that can stop a budding infection, such as E. coli. Antibiotics destroy both good and bad bacteria in the gut so, when taking them, eat plenty of yoghurt of counter this.

Recommended for:
digestive
stress
joints

Eggs

★★★★

Free-range eggs are free from unwanted chemicals and lower in cholesterol than battery-farmed eggs. For all but a tiny minority of people, the cholesterol in eggs does not affect blood cholesterol. Eggs are easily digested and supply protein, zinc, B vitamins, and other nutrients.

Recommended for:
stress
skin

Butter

★★★★

After many years of being told that margarine is better for you than butter, the tide has turned. Used modestly, butter is healthier than most margarines, which often contain artery-damaging trans-fats, and it's delicious too. Butter is virtually all fat, and 60 per cent of that is saturated fat. One hundred grams of butter provides 740 calories, but it also supplies vitamins A, D, and E. Salted butter may contain up to 1300mg of salt per 100g (3½oz); you can avoid this by simply choosing an unsalted variety. Under UK regulation, butter can be coloured but it may not contain antioxidants, unless the finished product is used exclusively for catering or manufacturing. It's best to choose uncoloured brands.

Be sparing with the butter and your food will taste better for it.

Recommended for:
fatigue
joints
skin

Cheese

★★★★

For thousands of years, cheese has been important for human nutrition. The ancient Greeks and Romans made cheese, and it was so much a part of the Roman diet that every Roman legionnaire was entitled to a daily portion.

We worry that so many young women avoid this vital source of bone-building calcium, protein, and vitamins A, B, and D. They do it in the pursuit of thinness, just because cheese contains some fat. Apart from calcium and vitamins, cheese also supplies some zinc in a form the body can easily use – 100g (3½oz) of cheese supplies one-quarter of the daily zinc requirement for adults. Cheese can benefit men, too – zinc is vital for normal male sexual function. Cheese is also good for children and adolescents, as they need the calcium for their developing bones. Worryingly, statistics indicate that around half of British youngsters aren't getting enough calcium in their diets.

People who get migraines may react badly to a chemical known as tyramine, which cheese contains and which can trigger migraine attacks. There are also people with an allergy to cow's milk. Goat's and sheep's cheeses make wonderful alternatives to cow's milk cheese and for both of these groups, they usually present no problems. Most goat's cheese is soft and mild. If you like hard cheese, Spanish Manchego is an exceptional one (made from sheep's milk) with a full but mild flavour. French Roquefort, Italian Pecorino, and Greek Feta are stronger sheep's cheeses.

● ●

Recommended for:
fatigue
stress

Beef and lamb

★★★★

These meats contain protein, iron, zinc, and B vitamins. Free-range cattle produce CLA, a unique fat that helps to control cholesterol and aids weight management. Beef and lamb from biologically reared livestock is much lower in saturated fat than intensively reared meat. This meat is also free of the chemical cocktail found in intensively reared meat, which includes hormones, antibiotics, pesticides, and insecticides. Excessive consumption of red meat is linked to bowel cancer, but three portions a week is fine.

Recommended for:
fatigue

Liver

★★★★

Liver is lovely and an amazing source of essential nutrients, but we don't eat enough of it these days. It supplies iron and zinc that can be easily absorbed, and is the richest dietary source of vitamins A and B12. It also contains other B vitamins. Don't eat liver, however, if you are, or are trying to become, pregnant as excessive vitamin A may cause birth defects; an average portion of liver provides five times your daily requirement of this nutrient.

Recommended for:
stress
fatigue

Chicken

★★★★

Free-range or organic chicken, like beef and lamb from biologically reared livestock, not only tastes better than the factory-farmed birds, but is also a great deal healthier. A properly reared chicken, without the antibiotics, growth hormones, and other unwanted chemicals poured down its throat from hatching to dispatching, will have a lower fat content than red meat or commercially produced chicken. Most of the fat will be in the skin and is easily removed. Because they are feeding on natural grasses, free-range chickens have more of the healthy omega-3 fatty acids and much less of the worst saturated fats than their commercially reared counterparts.

Free-range birds also build more muscle, and more muscle means more protein. In addition, they are an excellent source of B vitamins and of easily absorbed iron and zinc. And chicken soup is comforting as well as anti-viral.

• • • • • • • • • • • • • • • • • • •

Recommended for:
circulatory
stress

Oily fish

★★★★

Over the last hundred years, our consumption of fish has slowly declined, even as we've made more and more exciting discoveries about its nutritional role in our diets. Oily fish, in particular, is one of the richest known sources of a vital ingredient in human health – the essential fatty acid omega-3.

Professor Hugh Sinclair was the first person to recognise the importance of essential fatty acids, or EFAs. He wanted to know why the Inuit, who ate primarily whale blubber and fish (a diet which, according to the wisdom at that time, was high in saturated fats and therefore very heart-unfriendly), should have low levels of cardiovascular disease. There was one clue: the Inuit were known to bleed very easily. So Sinclair put himself on a diet of whale blubber for 100 days and at the end of the study, his platelet and cholesterol levels had gone down, and he too bled easily. An ingredient was thinning his blood. The secret ingredients, he eventually worked out, were the EFAs, and one in particular, called omega-3.

Historically, we have consumed a diet with equal levels of omega-3 and omega-6 fatty acids, but in the last century, as our diet has contained more vegetable oils and refined grains and less oily fish, the balance has been upset. The deficiency in omega-3 fatty acids may be partly responsible for soaring levels of depression, heart disease, and behavioural problems in the young, as well as a spectrum of illnesses. So remember to eat that oily fish!

There are two problems that complicate the issue further. The survival of some species is currently threatened, and certain fish should be eaten only rarely because they may be contaminated with pollution. Fortunately, the healthiest fish are less threatened: you can eat herring, mackerel, pilchards, sardines, sprats, trout (not farmed), whitebait, anchovies, and carp (farmed) without anxiety or guilt. Non-oily fish, Pacific cod, Dover sole, white bass, and Alaskan and Pacific halibut are all sustainably caught and good sources of protein.

• • • • • • • • • • • • • • • • • •

Recommended for:
circulatory
fatigue
joints

Molluscs

★★★★

These are the closed-shell seafoods, such as mussels, oysters, cockles, whelks, winkles, clams, and scallops. Molluscs, especially oysters, are an excellent source of zinc, which, together with cockles and whelks, contain as much iron as a fillet steak. Winkles are an even richer source of this essential mineral, supplying as much as the equivalent weight of liver.

Another good reason for eating molluscs is their high selenium content. This mineral is very deficient in the British diet, although it is less so in most parts of the US. Selenium deficiency has been closely linked with heart disease and considerably greater risks of cancer of the oesophagus and the prostate.

Casanova used to eat 70 oysters a day, and they have been a favourite aphrodisiac food for centuries, dating back to Roman times. What the Romans didn't know as they ate vast quantities of native Colchester oysters – the best in the world – was that they contained substantial quantities of zinc, an essential mineral for the production of sperm and the maintenance of male potency. A dozen of these magnificent molluscs provide more than you need for a whole week.

Molluscs should be eaten the day you buy them. The shells of all molluscs should be tightly closed before cooking. Many people are allergic to molluscs.

• •

Recommended for:
cancer
stress
fatigue

Crustaceans

★★★★

Crabs, lobsters, prawns, shrimps, crayfish, and langoustines are the most popular edible crustaceans. They provide the same amount of protein and other nutrients as white fish, although they are much saltier.

There has been controversy about the cholesterol content of crustaceans, but most experts believe that this is only a hazard if you have an inherited tendency to high cholesterol levels. Far from increasing the risk of heart disease, a regular intake of shellfish reduces levels of LDL (bad) fat, which are most dangerous. Crustaceans also contain valuable amounts of essential omega-3 fatty acids.

All crustaceans are highly nutritious alternatives to meat. They are excellent sources of protein, selenium, and tryptophan, and are very good sources of vitamins B12 and D. They also provide good amounts of minerals, including iron and zinc. Unfortunately, many people have an allergy to crustaceans. They also contain purines, which can aggravate gout.

Recommended for:
circulatory
stress
fatigue

Basil

★★★★

Basil is the traditional accompaniment to tomatoes in Mediterranean cookery and an ingredient of the green Italian pasta sauce pesto (pistou in Provence). Basil is both tonic and calming to the nervous system, making it a natural tranquillizer for the kind of frazzled nerves that lead to insomnia. If this is your problem, have a good "soupe au pistou" in the evening.

. . . .

Recommended for:
digestive
stress

Mint

★★★★

This popular herb comes in many varieties, and is often used for flavouring light summer dishes. Mint sauce with lamb was for a long time regarded by the French as culinary barbarism, but now they have acknowledged mint's beneficial effect on the digestion and have devised their own sauce paloise. Fragrant peppermint tea is a popular digestive throughout the Middle East. Mint also stimulates the heart and nerves. Drink this delicious tea instead of coffee for its mild lift.

. . . .

Recommended for:
circulatory
digestive

Oregano

★★★★

Oregano is the distinctive note in the smell of pizza. An obliging herb, it is almost as delicious dried as fresh. It is an effective antiseptic for the respiratory tract, so enjoy plenty of it in winter. It's also good for colic.

• •

Recommended for:
digestive
respiratory

Chives

★★★★

Chives share many of the healing properties of garlic and onions, which belong to the same family. They impart a milder flavour, however, so are good for flavouring delicate sauces. The pretty mauve flowers of chives can also be eaten, and look good when scattered on a summer salad.

• •

Recommended for:
cancer
circulatory

Sage
★★★★

Sage and onion stuffing for roast goose or turkey is true kitchen medicine, since sage aids the digestion of rich, heavy food. Italian cooks always add a leaf of sage to the pan when they fry sausages or pork.

Sage also acts as a stimulant to the central nervous system, making it a valuable tonic for convalescents or for those suffering from stress or nervous exhaustion. It is good for respiratory complaints, and the French make a tonic wine with it, which is admirable for those who are run down or are getting over a nasty viral infection.

Sage is powerful stuff, however – it can dry up mother's milk – so don't use it medicinally for more than a week at a time.

Recommended for:
digestive
stress
respiratory

Marjoram

★★★★

Sweet or pot marjoram is the gentler garden variety of wild marjoram or oregano (*p.97*), which grows on the hillsides of Greece. In medieval times, sweet marjoram was an important household herb and was used to scent rooms and as a furniture polish.

Unsurprisingly, perhaps, marjoram and oregano have similar properties. Sweet marjoram is particularly valued for its calming qualities, and the essential oil is strongly sedative. The leaves can be used to make a soothing tea, or they can be chopped finely and added as a flavouring to salads, sauces, and other dishes.

Recommended for:
digestive
stress

Parsley

★★★★

Parsley is rich in vitamins A and C and in iron, calcium, and potassium, as well as in life-giving chlorophyll. Use it fresh and use it lavishly.

Herbalists value parsley for its diuretic action, and parsley tea was used in the trenches in World War I for soldiers suffering from kidney complications following dysentery. It also helps to eliminate uric acid, making it useful in the treatment of rheumatism and gout. Parsley tea was an old country aid to digestion: Maurice Messegué recalls the monster pot brewed by his grandmother Sophie after a Lucullan feast of foie gras, roast chicken, sautéed mushrooms, crêpes, custards, and apple tart.

Add a bunch of fresh parsley whenever you make a freshly pressed vegetable juice to enjoy the full benefits of this important herb.

● ● ● ● ● ● ● ● ● ● ● ● ● ● ● ● ● ● ● ●

Recommended for:
digestive
joints
urinary

Rosemary

★★★★

Rosemary originated in the hot, dry climate of the Mediterranean countries, where it has long been an important medicinal and household herb. We know it mainly as the inseparable companion of roast lamb and chicken in Mediterranean cookery. It is once more a powerful friend to the digestive system, prompting the production of extra bile for fat digestion.

"Rosemary for remembrance" is an old adage, and it's true that rosemary also stimulates the adrenal cortex. Rosemary wine, in small doses, is valuable in states of general debility, including loss of memory, strain, and nervous tension.

• • • • • • • • • • • • • • • • • •

Recommended for:
digestive
stress

Savory

★★★★

Savory is one of the oldest herbs used for flavouring, and the ancient Romans often used it in sauces. The German name of this peppery little plant means "bean-herb", since it eases the digestion of this challenging food. Try it with split peas, broad beans, and lentils too. It benefits the entire digestive tract and has an antiseptic action on the gut.

Recommended for:
digestive

Fennel

★★★★

The dark green fronds of fennel are a classic ingredient of the court-bouillon for fish dishes and soups. You can also add them to mayonnaise to serve with cold fish in summer. Fennel goes particularly well with rich fish such as mackerel. An excellent aid to digestion, it prevents wind or colic.

Recommended for:
digestive

Tarragon

★★★★

Tho dolioato, distinctive flavour of this herb seems particularly French. Tarragon is often used with roast chicken, in sauces, in omelettes, or to flavour a wine vinegar. The dried herb, however, is a pale shadow of the fresh. Tarragon can help relieve wind, flatulence, and acidity.

Recommended for:
digestive

Thyme

★★★★

Thyme contributes to the deepest aromatic note in a bouquet garni, and it would be hard to imagine a robust peasant daube of beef, or a springtime lamb stew, without this herb. Its medicinal qualities are just as impressive. Thyme is a powerful antiseptic as well as a general stimulant to the body's natural resistance, with marked antiviral and antibacterial activity. It is also a tonic to the nervous system.

Recommended for:
stress
respiratory

Dill
★★★★

Both the ancient Egyptians and the Greeks valued dill for its medicinal properties and used it to treat indigestion and other stomach complaints. The leaves, flowers, and seeds of this pretty, feathery herb are all useful in cooking, and the seeds are still sometimes served as a digestive following a rich meal. Dill is a favourite accompaniment to fish in Scandinavia, and it is particularly good with salmon, whether fresh or smoked. Dried dill is a piquant addition to bland cheeses or to salad dressings.

Babies may first taste dill in the form of gripe water, where it is highly effective; in fact its name comes from an Anglo-Saxon word meaning "to lull".

Recommended for:
digestive
stress

Dandelion

★★★★

The bitter taste of dandelion leaves is a clue to their usefulness: they have a long-standing reputation in the treatment of liver problems. Juice from the roots could be found at every apothecary for centuries. A digestive and urinary system tonic, dandelion is also a gentle, effective diuretic, helping to eliminate uric acid, excess cholesterol, and urea. The plant supplies enough potassium to compensate for the amount lost in the urine. It is also known as a blood-cleanser and is helpful for toxic or inflammatory conditions of the skin or joints.

The leaves are nearly as useful as the root. They are rich in vitamins A and C, beta-carotene, and chlorophyll, and the iron that they supply is more readily taken up by the body than the iron in spinach. Add the young leaves – the older leaves are too bitter   to any mixed green salad and enjoy an all-round tonic.

Recommended for:
circulatory
digestive
fatigue
joints
urinary

Bay leaves

★★★★

The distinctive flavour of bay leaves is an intrinsic part of the classic French bouquet garni (a bunch of herbs used to flavour slowly cooked dishes). Bay leaves are prized for their antiseptic properties and for their assistance to the digestion, helping to ward off wind and cramps.

· ·

Recommended for:
digestive
respiratory

Juniper

★★★★

These tiny berries are responsible for giving gin its unique flavour. They impart a powerful tang when used in cooking. Herbalists use them as a diuretic and to help clear excess uric acid from the body. Like so many culinary herbs, they are also a tonic to the digestive system.

· ·

Recommended for:
digestive
urinary

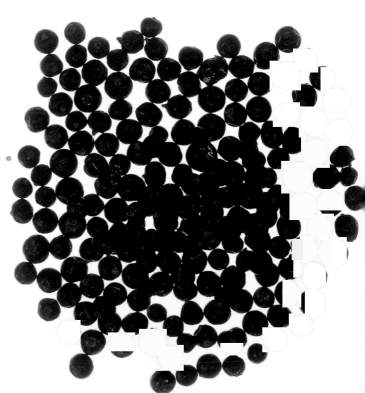

Nutmeg

★★★★

This spice, familiar from so many favourite winter sweet treats, can have a mildly uplifting effect in small doses and is also good for the digestion. Don't overdo it, though, because it can be hallucinogenic in large quantities.

. . . .

Recommended for:
digestive
stress

Cinnamon

★★★★

This excellent spice lends its delicate but distinctive flavour to dozens of minced meat and other dishes in Middle Eastern cookery. In Northern Europe it's one of the warming winter favourites used in festive puddings or mulled wine. Cinnamon is a potent antiseptic. It is also a tonic and a stimulant, warming the whole system and helping to combat the fatigue and listlessness that so often attend bouts of flu or other viral infections. Add a stick to the hot, sweet toddy you take to bed at the start of a cold.

. . . .

Recommended for:
digestive
respiratory

Chilli peppers

★★★★

These small, hot peppers are used fresh,
or dried in the form of chilli powder
or cayenne pepper. Chillis are popular
wherever people like their food with a
real kick to it. Nineteenth-century herbalists
had boundless faith in the life-saving and
restorative powers of chilli or cayenne
pepper. They used teaspoon doses for
typhoid and cholera patients in extremis.
Research has confirmed the chilli
pepper's beneficent effect on the heart
and circulatory system. A shot of chilli or
cayenne added to a hot drink is a sure boost
to a sluggish digestion. Scientists have found
that certain pungent foods, such as mustard,
horseradish, chilli, and garlic, contain
constituents called mucokinetic agents that
help shift excess mucus from the lungs, so
that it can be coughed up. Thus chillis and
their derivatives also have a tonic effect
on the respiratory system.

• •

Recommended for:
circulatory
digestive
respiratory

Caraway

★★★★

A spice whose use dates from ancient times, caraway has been found in ancient Egyptian tombs and is mentioned in the Bible. Although it has long been popular in the cold northern European countries, caraway is also used in Indian cuisine, where the seeds are served as a digestive after the meal. Similarly, in Central Europe, caraway seeds are a well known aid to digestion – people often chew a few of them before sitting down to a rich meal. They are particularly effective for coping with wind or flatulence (as is dill, which contains the same compound, carvone). Add caraway seeds to potentially "windy" dishes, such as cabbage or beans.

● ● ● ● ● ● ● ● ● ● ● ● ● ● ● ●

Recommended for:
digestive

Cloves

★★★★

Cloves come from a tropical evergreen tree and have been important in European culture ever since the spice routes opened up in the Middle Ages. The spiky whole cloves are actually dried, unopened flower buds. They have been used for centuries for purposes as diverse as flavouring foods, treating toothache, and freshening the breath.

Like cinnamon, cloves are both powerfully antiseptic and a warming boost to the circulation. They are used in much the same way as cinnamon, and like that spice, they can be added to dishes whole or can be ground into a powder first. Try adding a bruised clove or two to any herbal tea to provide an extra lift.

Recommended for:
digestive
stress
respiratory

Cumin

★★★★

People often associate cumin with Indian curries, but the incomparable smell given off by the warmed, crushed seeds evokes Middle Eastern cookery, too. Cumin is also an important flavouring in Mexican cuisine and is an essential ingredient in many Mexican dishes. Like so many herbs and spices, cumin has a soothing effect on the digestive system, which is probably why it is mixed with yoghurt to make the cooling lassi drinks of Indian cuisine.

Use cumin in rich fried dishes or with beans to counter flatulence and dyspepsia. It has a special affinity with lamb dishes.

Recommended for:
digestive

Coriander

★★★★

Coriander is mentioned in Sanskrit writings and in the Bible. It was introduced into Europe by the ancient Romans, who found it useful as a preservative for meat. Today, we know coriander seed as an essential ingredient of curry powders. It is also added to cold starters cooked *à la grecque*. Powdered coriander seed adds a distinctive North African flavour to meat and fish dishes. In hot, stimulating food, this mild spice is valued for its cooling quality and its assistance to the digestion.

The chopped leaves also have a delicious, piquant flavour and are good added to a plain green salad. The fresh leaves also go well with cold cooked chicken.

Recommended for:
digestive

Garlic

★★★★

The word garlic comes from two Anglo-Saxon words that together mean "spear leek". This name probably derived from the shape of the garlic plant's leaves, which are sharp and pointed.

Garlic is yet another food that was introduced to Britain by the Romans. The Roman soldiers used to put cloves of garlic between their toes in order to prevent fungal infections of the feet. In Britain, the plant was established in the wild from the cloves that dropped to the ground.

Garlic is not only a delicious flavouring for food, but it also has many health-giving properties. From ancient times right up to the end of the nineteenth century, garlic was the most frequently used medicinal plant throughout the world. All sorts of diseases and conditions, including bronchitis, asthma, indigestion, gout, and even (as the Romans apparently knew) athlete's foot, can be helped by garlic. It has antiviral, antibacterial, and antifungal properties, with virtually no side effects apart from irritation of the gut in some sensitive people.

The most exciting discovery about garlic so far, however, has been its effect on the heart and circulation. Like its close relative the onion (*p.58*), garlic has the ability to thin the blood. It contains the sulphur compound allicin, which helps the body eliminate cholesterol and also reduces the amount of unhealthy fats produced by the liver.

When, in studies, garlic was given to healthy volunteers who were fed diets rich in fatty foods, garlic reduced blood cholesterol by up to 15 per cent. In another study, people with high cholesterol levels who took garlic supplements – but did not otherwise change their diets – reduced their cholesterol levels by an average of 12 per cent over a four-month period.

Recommended for:
circulatory
digestive
joints

the superfoods 115

Ginger

★★★★

Ginger is another warming, antiseptic spice. It is widely used in the cookery of meat and fish in the East, where it helps counter putrefaction. It is equally popular as a sweet spice in the West. It is the tuberous root of a perennial plant found in tropical regions and should be peeled before slicing or grating.

It's far better to use the fresh root wherever possible, since dried ginger is poor stuff by comparison. Ginger aids digestion and is unexpectedly useful against nausea. In fact, clinical trials have shown it to be more effective than the standard drugs against motion sickness. Another benefit is that it has none of the side effects of conventional anti-nausea drugs, and pregnant women and children can use it safely. Fresh ginger grated into hot lemon and honey as a bedtime drink can stop a cold or chill in its tracks.

• • • • • • • • • • • • • • • • • • •

Recommended for:
digestive
joints

Horseradish

★★★★

Horseradish was originally a medicinal herb, but these days most of us know it only as a condiment made up in jars and eaten as a flavouring with roast beef. It deserves to be used more adventurously: try the fresh root grated into salad dressing, mayonnaise, or cottage cheese, or try adding a little horseradish to some natural yoghurt as a tangy accompaniment to smoked fish.

Horseradish is an invigorating herb and is powerfully stimulant to the digestion, which is a reason for eating it with rich foods, such as roast beef or oily fish. It also clears excess catarrh and counters infection. Since the volatile oil that gives horseradish its flavour is destroyed by heat, the herb should only be added fresh to food after cooking.

• • • • • • • • • • • • • • • • • •

Recommended for:
digestive

Brewer's yeast

★★★★

Although it is no longer quite the healthfood shop star of former days, brewer's yeast is still an unrivalled source of the B-complex vitamins, which serves many purposes: it helps to break down carbohydrates, proteins, and fats and supports the nervous system, among other functions. With particularly high levels of iron, zinc, manganese, magnesium, and potassium, brewer's yeast supplies protein, and is also high in chromium, which has been shown to help lower cholesterol and reduce blood sugar levels. It is rich in the nucleic acid RNA, which is vital to the immune system.

On its own, brewer's yeast does not taste agreeable, but spooned into your morning smoothie and blended with milk, yoghurt, and fruit juices, with a little honey, it registers as a pleasant, nutty flavour.

Since brewer's yeast is high in purines, it should be avoided by people with gout.

• • • • • • • • • • • • • • • • • • •

Recommended for:
circulatory
stress
fatigue

Oils

★★★★

Olive oil Like all cold-pressed vegetable oils, extra-virgin olive oil is extracted from the olives without the use of heat or chemicals, resulting in the purest possible finished product. Olive oil is the best digested of vegetable oils and provides the strongest stimulation of the gallbladder, an aid to all fat digestion.

Just two tablespoons of extra-virgin olive oil provides almost 90 per cent of monounsaturated fat and nearly 20 per cent of the vitamin E that you need for a whole day. The monounsaturated fats in olive oil help reduce cholesterol levels, and the oil acts as a strong antioxidant as well due to its high vitamin E content, protecting cells from damage. Some of the natural chemicals in olive oil prevent the absorption of cholesterol and increase the level of HDL (good) fat in the bloodstream. One study showed that adding two tablespoons of olive oil to the daily diet with no other dietary changes produced a significant fall in cholesterol levels.

Flaxseed oil Cold-pressed flaxseed oil is extremely rich in omega-3 fatty acids, especially alphalinolenic acid (ALA). Some people believe that flaxseed oil is as healthy as fish oils, as the ALA can be converted in the body into EPA – eicosapentaenoic acid. Not all people produce the enzyme necessary for this to happen, however. ALA is important as a balance to omega-6 fatty acids in the diet. Flaxseed oil turns rancid if exposed to heat, light, or air. Keep it in the refrigerator and use it well before its sell by date. It's not suitable for frying or cooking, but it's perfect added to dressings, sauces, and marinades.

Recommended for:
cancer
circulatory

Honey

★★★★

Ancient societies used honey for energy and sweetening and as a preservative. To this day, milk and honey is a popular bedtime remedy for insomnia.

Traditionally, honey has been valued for both internal and external medicine, relieving coughs, stomachache, indigestion, and injuries. New Zealand Manuka honey is now widely used in hospitals as a sterile dressing for plastic surgery wounds and severe ulceration. It kills most bacteria, including the dreaded MRSA.

Recommended for:
digestive
fatigue
respiratory

Molasses

★★★★

Molasses is the last extract from sugar cane when the sugar is refined out of it. Weight for weight, crude black molasses contains more calcium than milk, more iron than eggs – three milligrams in one tablespoon – and a very high level of potassium. It is also rich in many B vitamins. Its flavour is quite powerful. Molasses should not be eaten straight from the spoon as a matter of habit, however, because of its high sugar content – a risk to teeth and gums.

Recommended for:
stress
fatigue
joints

Chocolate

★★★★

When the famous botanist Linnaeus came to name the cocoa tree, he called it *theobroma*, which means "food of the gods". He had good reason for this – a major constituent of the bean is a chemical called theobromine, which acts in the brain to trigger the release of natural feel-good chemicals called endorphins. These chemicals kindle feelings of romance, love, and arousal, and combat depression. Chocolate also contains caffeine, which is a stimulant that makes chocolate a mild diuretic.

Dark chocolate contains fat and provides 500 calories per 100g (3½oz) serving. However, it also supplies iron, magnesium, useful amounts of protein, and traces of some other minerals, as well as some B vitamins. You'll need to do two hours of brisk walking, ride your bike for an hour and a half, or swim non-stop for a full hour to burn off a large chocolate bar.

● ● ● ● ● ● ● ● ● ● ● ● ● ● ● ● ●

Recommended for:
stress

Beer
★★★★

Beer is one of the best nutritional sources of silicon, which is essential for bones. As little as half a pint a day could help prevent osteoporosis, which causes more than 200,000 fractures every year, most of them in women.

There's more good news about beer, as recent research reveals that the hops used in traditional brewing are a good source of phytoestrogens, which are natural plant hormones that protect against osteoporosis. If you really want strong bones, next time you have a pub lunch order a ploughman's and a glass of beer. The calcium in the cheese and the phytoestrogens in the beer are perfect bone-builders.

Beer is also rich in vitamins B6 and B12 and folic acid, which many women lack in their diets. As a bonus, hops have a natural antibiotic action that kills the *Helicobacter pylori* bacterium, which is the cause of most gastric ulcers. With lots of potassium but little sodium, sensible quantities of beer can be good for blood pressure.

Recommended for:
circulatory
digestive

Red wine

In most parts of the world, the drinker's toast is to their companion's good health – "à votre santé","salud", "skoal", "prost", "l'chayim" – and there are indeed some health benefits in drinking red wine. It's one of the factors in the Mediterranean diet that is known to protect against heart disease. Research done in France shows that men who drink moderate amounts of red wine regularly have a 30 per cent lower risk of death from all causes than either men who drink heavily or those who abstain from alcohol completely. This may be due at least in part to the natural antioxidants, known as phenolic compounds, that red grapes contain. These phenolic compounds are known to protect against heart and circulatory disease.

People who drink white wine in moderation may also be improving their health, as studies done in the US show that white wine drinkers have the healthiest lungs.

Recommended for:
circulatory
respiratory

Tea
★★★★

Nutritionally, tea contains very little in terms of vitamins and minerals. The leaves do contain tannins, which are good for eye problems – a used teabag dipped in cold water and placed over closed eyes for 10 minutes gives instant relief for sticky, itchy, and tired eyes.

By far the most exciting benefits of tea come from the bioflavonoids it contains. These natural plant chemicals, which act as antioxidants, neutralize the damaging free radicals that cause heart and circulatory problems. Two to four cups of tea a day are necessary for this extra protection, and although green tea is richer in protective substances, British brew also contains significant amounts. Green tea is the most cancer-protective of all teas.

Tea can even help concentration, and it's not the caffeine. There's another ingredient that helps concentration and speeds up the learning process, but we don't yet know what it is.

• • • • • • • • • • • • • • • • • •

Recommended for:
cancer
circulatory

Coffee

Coffee is known for containing caffeine, but there's also caffeine in tea, chocolate, and cola drinks. On the positive side, caffeine stimulates the brain, aids concentration, and fights fatigue. Surprisingly, coffee may also help some people with asthma, it increases the potency of painkillers, and may even improve migraine.

On the other hand, coffee can increase blood pressure in non-regular users by 10 per cent for three hours after consumption. Too much coffee is addictive. It is also linked to PMS, cyclical breast lumps, poor fertility, and low birth weight in babies.

Caffeine adversely affects the body's absorption of the minerals iron and zinc, so pregnant women and vegetarians should reduce the amount of coffee they drink. Coffee also stimulates the production of stomach acid, which can lead to heartburn and indigestion.

It's fine to enjoy a cup of good coffee, a pot of fragrant tea, or a mug of soothing cocoa, but limit the amount you drink to avoid caffeine addiction.

Recommended for:
fatigue
respiratory

126

Recipes

Pumpkin soup serves 4

DIGESTIVE · RESPIRATORY · SKIN

750g (1½lb) piece of pumpkin
1tsp olive oil
1 large onion, sliced
1 clove garlic, chopped
1 bay leaf
750ml (1¼pt) vegetable stock
   (*p.188*)
2 carrots, finely grated
2tbs parsley, chopped
wholemeal garlic
   croutons (*p.188*)

Cut the pumpkin into wedges, skin and all, remove seeds and save them, put the pumpkin in an ovenproof dish, and bake for half an hour at 140°C (270°F/gas 1). Drain off the surplus water, which you save, and remove the skin. Heat the oil in a heavy-bottomed pan and sweat the onion, the garlic, and the bay leaf for a few minutes over a gentle heat. Add the stock, pumpkin and its water, and simmer for 30 minutes. Stir in the grated carrots, add the chopped parsley, check the seasoning, and serve with the croutons.

Onion soup serves 4

CIRCULATORY · RESPIRATORY · URINARY

2 large onions
1tbs oil
900ml (1½pt) vegetable stock
   (*p.188*)
fresh thyme
black pepper
½tsp salt-free yeast extract
4 slices wholemeal bread
125g (4oz) grated Cheddar
   cheese

Peel and slice the onions, heat the oil in a heavy-bottomed pan, and sweat the onions until slightly golden. Add the stock, thyme, pepper, and yeast extract, bring to the boil, and simmer gently for 15–20 minutes. Pour the soup into flameproof bowls, if you have them, float the bread on top, sprinkle grated cheese on top of the bread, and put under a hot grill until melted.

Spanish white garlic soup serves 4

CANCER · CIRCULATORY · JOINTS · RESPIRATORY

175g (6oz) almonds, blanched
   or ground
4 big cloves garlic, crushed
1 thick slice white bread,
   soaked in water and
   squeezed dry
100ml (3fl oz) olive oil
100ml (3fl oz) iced water
a little lemon juice
salt
a few peeled Muscat grapes,
   if in season

If you have fresh almonds, soak them in tepid water for 10 minutes, then the skins will slip off easily. Whole almonds should be ground in a food processor or coffee mill. Add the garlic and the bread to the ground almonds, and process thoroughly until smooth. Then add the olive oil drop by drop, as for a mayonnaise. Add the iced water until the soup is a thick cream. Add lemon juice, and salt to taste.

Traditionally this soup is served with a few peeled white Muscat grapes floating in it.

Borscht serves 4

CANCER · FATIGUE

500g (1lb) raw beetroot
30g (1oz) butter
1tbs olive oil
1 medium-sized onion, sliced
2 carrots, peeled and sliced
2 sticks celery, chopped
1 small bulb fennel, chopped
1.2litre (2pt) vegetable
   stock (p.188)
1tsp fresh thyme, chopped
1tbs fresh parsley, chopped
1 bay leaf
salt and pepper
juice of 1 lemon
1-2tbs natural yoghurt
wholemeal croutons (p.188)

Peel the beetroot and slice into thin strips. Heat the butter and oil in a heavy bottomed pan, sweat the onion, then add the beetroot and the carrot, celery, and fennel. Sauté over a very low heat for a few minutes, and then add the stock and the herbs. Bring to the boil, turn the heat down, and simmer until the vegetables are soft   about 30 minutes.

Strain into another pan, purée the vegetables in a blender or food processor, return them to the soup, add the lemon juice, and seasoning to taste. Serve with a swirl of natural yoghurt in each bowl, and wholemeal croutons.

Carrot soup serves 4 ▶

CIRCULATORY · RESPIRATORY · SKIN

375g (12oz) old carrots
1 small onion
1tbs olive oil
600ml (1pt) vegetable stock
   (*p.188*)
juice of 3 oranges, and grated
   rind of 1 orange
a sprig of fresh mint
150g (5oz) natural yoghurt

Clean and coarsely grate the carrots; clean and finely chop the onion. Heat the oil in a heavy-bottomed saucepan, add the carrots and onion, and cook very gently until the carrots are soft and mushy. Pour on the stock, add the mint, and leave to simmer for 20 minutes. Blend or liquidize, add the orange juice, and season to taste. Serve hot or cold with yoghurt and sprinkled with the grated orange rind.

Jerusalem artichoke soup serves 4

JOINTS · SKIN · CIRCULATORY · FATIGUE

1tbs vegetable oil
500g (1lb) Jerusalem
   artichokes, thoroughly
   washed and sliced
1 medium-sized onion, finely
   chopped
900ml (1½pt) vegetable stock
   (*p.188*)
1 small bunch watercress,
   washed and trimmed
wholemeal garlic croutons
   (*p.188*)
2tbs fresh parsley, finely
   chopped
a little cream, if desired

Heat the oil, add the artichokes and onion, and sauté until the onion is just transparent, but not browned. Add the vegetable stock and simmer until the artichoke pieces are soft and tender. Put in a liquidizer or blender, together with the watercress, return to the pan, and reheat. Serve piping hot with wholemeal garlic croutons and sprinkled with chopped parsley. Add a swirl of cream for luxury.

Brown rice and celery soup serves 4

CANCER · DIGESTIVE · FATIGUE · JOINTS · URINARY

1litre (1¾pt) vegetable stock
(*p.188*)
4 sticks celery, cleaned and
diced
2tbs olive oil
1 medium-sized onion,
finely chopped
30g (2oz) brown rice, washed
and drained
salt and pepper
1tbs fresh parsley, chopped

Put the stock in a pan, add the diced celery, bring to the boil and simmer until the celery is soft. Strain off the stock and reserve. Purée the softened celery in a food processor or blender. In a clean pan, heat the oil, melt the onion; when it is transparent, add the rice, stir it around; add the celery purée, the vegetable stock, and season with salt and pepper to taste. Bring to the boil, and simmer until the rice is cooked through – about 35 minutes. Sprinkle with the parsley.

Verdant broth serves 4

CANCER · CIRCULATORY · JOINTS · SKIN · RESPIRATORY

1 fat leek, washed, trimmed,
and sliced
1 head celery, washed,
trimmed, and sliced
1litre (1¾pt) water
1tbs olive oil
1 large onion, sliced
1 bunch watercress
1 bunch parsley
1tbs olive oil
salt and pepper
wholemeal garlic
croutons (*p.188*)

Boil the water in a large pan. Put the cleaned green top of the leek and the top and tough outer leaves of the celery into the boiling water to make a stock. Simmer for 30 minutes, then discard the vegetables. Heat the oil, sauté the finely sliced white part of the leek and the sliced onion until translucent, but don't let them brown. Add the sliced celery and the stock, season with salt and pepper to taste, and simmer for half an hour. Then put in the food processor together with the watercress and parsley, both carefully cleaned. Serve this fresh-tasting broth with garlic croutons.

Sweetcorn and haddock chowder serves 4

2tbs sunflower oil

90g (3oz) streaky bacon, cut into strips

1 onion, chopped

1 bay leaf

a sprig of fresh thyme

2 medium-sized potatoes, peeled and diced

375g (12oz) tin of sweetcorn, drained

300ml (½pt) milk

300ml (½pt) buttermilk

150ml (¼pt) water

250g (8oz) undyed smoked haddock, cut into 2.5cm (1in) cubes, skinned and boned

1tbs fresh chives, chopped

salt and pepper

This is a one-pot meal. Keep the cooking time short by cutting the potatoes small so that they cook through in 10 minutes. Ideally they should crumble and thicken the soup.

Heat the oil, and fry the bacon until crisp. Remove and reserve. Fry the onion until softened but not brown, add the bay leaf, thyme, potato, sweetcorn, milk, buttermilk, and water. Simmer for 10 minutes, add the fish and chives, and simmer gently for a further 5 minutes. Season to taste with salt and pepper, and serve with the strips of bacon arranged over the top.

Oats and broccoli pottage serves 4

CANCER · CIRCULATORY

1tbs olive oil

6 spring onions, chopped

500g (1lb) broccoli florets

60g (2oz) porridge oats

1litre (1¾pt) half milk and half vegetable stock (*p.188*)

freshly ground pepper

freshly ground nutmeg

1tbs single cream

1tbs fresh chives, chopped

Heat the oil and sweat the onions until they are soft. Add the broccoli and stir for a couple of minutes. Add the oats, and stir for another minute or two. Slowly add the milk and stock, stirring. Cover and simmer very gently for 10 minutes. Season with a little freshly ground pepper and nutmeg. Just before serving the soup, stir in the cream and sprinkle with the chopped chives.

Asparagus citronette serves 4 ▶

DIGESTIVE · URINARY

500g (1lb) asparagus
3tbs extra-virgin olive oil
juice of a big lemon
black pepper

Wash the asparagus thoroughly and trim off the tough bottoms of the stalks: do not discard these, as you can use them for soup together with the asparagus cooking water. An asparagus steamer gives the best results, but failing that, cook them lying flat in boiling water in a deep, wide frying pan – or even a wok. They are done when you can easily pierce the fleshiest part of the stems with a knife. Drain – saving the water – and set aside to cool. To make the dressing, combine the oil, lemon juice, and pepper in a jug.

NOTE: To make asparagus soup from the stock and trimmings, put the cut-off ends – all but the really dirty ones – into the cooking water. Add 2-3 small, peeled potatoes and 1 whole spear of asparagus. Bring to the boil, simmer until the potatoes are done, liquidize, and serve with a swirl of low-fat natural yoghurt.

Classic crudités serves 4

CANCER · DIGESTIVE · FATIGUE · RESPIRATORY · SKIN

6-10 radishes, washed
2 carrots, peeled
4-6 young beetroots,
   washed
2-3 sticks celery, washed
juice of half a lemon
1tbs olive oil
1tbs fresh parsley, chopped

In French restaurants, crudités can run to a dozen different dishes. The classics are fresh radishes with their green tops; raw carrots, peeled and grated; grated raw young beetroot; and chunks of crisp celery. All of these may be served with a lemon and olive oil dressing, with a sprinkling of fresh parsley on top.

Tomato and herb omelette serves 1 ▶

DIGESTIVE · FATIGUE · RESPIRATORY

1 medium-sized tomato
1tbs olive oil
3 free-range eggs
2tbs fresh herbs, chopped –
   parsley, chives, chervil
salt and pepper

Omelettes are best made one at a time, although two people can share a big one. These quantities make one good-sized omelette, for 2 people, you can double the quantities, but use 5 rather than 6 eggs.

Skin the tomato – dip it in boiling water for a couple of minutes, then the skin slides off easily. Chop it. Beat the eggs in a bowl, then add the chopped tomatoes, the herbs – save a sprinkle for garnishing – and seasoning. Have a hot plate ready. Heat the oil. When it is sizzling hot, tip in the egg mixture. With a fork, keep lifting the edges so that the uncooked egg on top can run underneath. The whole operation should take less than a minute, and the egg should still be slightly runny on top when you roll the omelette out onto the plate. Sprinkle with the remaining herbs and serve at once.

Eggs with smoked haddock serves 2

CIRCULATORY · FATIGUE

175g (6oz) smoked haddock –
   avoid the lurid yellow kind
150ml (¼pt) milk
4 free-range eggs
freshly ground black pepper
1tbs butter

Cook the haddock in the milk for 2–3 minutes, then strain and save the milk. Flake the haddock, discarding skin and bones, and keep it hot. Beat the eggs with 2 tablespoons of the fishy milk, and season with a little pepper, but don't add salt. Melt the butter in a non-stick pan. Add the eggs, and stir briskly off the heat. Just before the eggs set, add the flaked haddock and stir it in. Serve with hot wholewheat toast. If you wish to serve 4 people, simply double the quantities.

Tuna and fennel pasta serves 4

CIRCULATORY · FATIGUE · JOINTS · SKIN · URINARY

200g (7oz) tuna, tinned in oil
1 large fennel bulb
1 tbs olive oil
2 cloves garlic, chopped
125ml (4fl oz) vegetable stock
   (*p.188*)
375g (12oz) spaghettini

Drain the oil from the tuna. Clean the fennel, chop up, including most of the feathery fronds, and mince in a food processor. Heat the oil in a saucepan, add the garlic and minced fennel, and fry gently until soft. Flake in the tuna, add the vegetable stock, and heat through. Meanwhile, cook the spaghettini in lots of boiling water until *al dente* (just tender). Drain, and quickly toss in the hot fennel and tuna sauce.

Red and yellow eggs serves 2

FATIGUE · URINARY

1 large red pepper
1 large yellow pepper
1 medium-sized onion
3–4 ripe red tomatoes
60g (2oz) butter
6 free-range eggs
salt and freshly ground
   black pepper
1 tbs fresh parsley, chopped

Halve the peppers, remove the ribs and seeds, and slice into fat strips. Finely chop the onion. Skin and roughly chop the tomatoes. Heat the butter in a non-stick pan. Add the peppers and onion and stew gently, covered, until they are softened, or for about 10 minutes. Stir in the tomatoes, and cook for about another 5 minutes. Beat the eggs, season with salt and pepper, and add the parsley. Add to the vegetable mixture, and stir until the eggs are just set.

Tuna and black olive sauce serves 4

CIRCULATORY · JOINTS

Tomato sauce (*p.180*)
200g (7oz) tuna, tinned in oil
8-10 pitted black olives
salt and pepper
250g (8oz) pasta, any shape

Make the tomato sauce. Add the tuna, drained of its oil, and the olives. Season to taste with salt and pepper, and heat through. Meanwhile, cook the pasta in a large pot of boiling water until *al dente* (just tender). Drain the pasta, stir in the sauce, and serve.

Eggs tonnato serves 4

CIRCULATORY · FATIGUE

4 free-range eggs
200g (7oz) tuna, tinned in oil
6tbs mayonnaise
1 small onion, finely chopped
2tbs fresh parsley, chopped
salt and pepper

This can be either a substantial starter or a light meal in itself. In the latter case, you may wish to use a few more eggs.

Hard-boil the eggs for 10 minutes. Peel the eggs, halve them, and arrange them face-down in a flat salad bowl. Drain the tuna, flake it, and add to the mayonnaise. Stir in the onion and 1 tablespoon of the parsley – save a little to garnish. Season to taste with salt and pepper. Spoon the mayonnaise over the eggs, and sprinkle with the rest of the parsley.

Pasta pesto with vegetables serves 4 ▶

CIRCULATORY · DIGESTIVE · STRESS · FATIGUE

1 tsp salt
300g (10oz) spaghetti
60g (2oz) French beans,
    cleaned and finely chopped
60g (2oz) new potatoes,
    peeled and finely diced
60g (2oz) courgettes, cleaned
    and diced
2–3 tbs pesto sauce
a few fresh basil leaves
Parmesan cheese, grated

To prepare the sauce, you can use ready-made pesto, available in jars.

Heat a large pan of water. When it boils, add the salt, and plunge in the spaghetti and the vegetables. By the time the pasta is cooked *al dente* (just tender), the vegetables should also be just tender. Just before you drain the spaghetti, take a tablespoon of the cooking water and stir it into the pesto. Drain the pasta and vegetables, and quickly transfer them to a hot dish. Stir in the pesto and toss. Garnish with the basil leaves and serve. Have a little grated Parmesan cheese ready for those who want it.

Tagliatelle with artichokes serves 4

CANCER · DIGESTIVE · FATIGUE · SKIN · URINARY

2 tbs butter
1 medium-sized onion,
    finely chopped
1 tbs plain flour
glass of dry white wine
1 425g (14oz) tin or jar of
    artichoke hearts, quartered
2 tbs fresh parsley, chopped
2 heaped tbs of grated
    Parmesan
500g (1lb) tagliatelle or
    other pasta

Traditionally, this recipe is made with fresh baby artichokes, but it can also be made with artichoke hearts packed in oil and sold in jars.

Heat the butter in a large saucepan and melt the onion without browning it. Add the flour and stir vigorously for 1–2 minutes. Drizzle in the wine and carry on stirring. Add the artichoke hearts and parsley, simmer, covered, until heated through – about 5 minutes. Add half the cheese, mix thoroughly, and keep warm. Boil a large pan of water and cook the pasta until *al dente* (just tender). Drain the pasta and put it in a large heated dish. Add the sauce, stir through quickly, and serve with the rest of the Parmesan.

Spaghetti con aglio e olio serves 4

CIRCULATORY · JOINTS · URINARY · FATIGUE

4tbs extra-virgin olive oil
3 cloves garlic, chopped
½tsp dried red chilli pepper,
    finely chopped
pinch of salt
500g (1lb) spaghetti or
    spaghettini
2 heaped tbs parsley, chopped

Heat the olive oil in a small pan and sauté the garlic and the chilli pepper until the garlic is just beginning to change colour. Turn off the heat and add a little salt. Put a big serving dish to warm. Cook the pasta in plenty of well-salted, boiling water. Stir occasionally and cook until the pasta is *al dente* (just tender). Drain, turn into the warmed serving dish, and add the sauce. Sprinkle the parsley over, toss, and serve immediately.

Green pasta salad serves 4

CANCER · CIRCULATORY · JOINTS · RESPIRATORY · SKIN

2 very young, tender
    courgettes
4 spring onions
250g (8oz) green fusilli or
    any other green pasta
handful of mangetout peas
3-5 baby sweetcorns
2tbs fresh parsley, chopped
3tbs extra-virgin olive oil
juice of a large lemon
seasoning to taste
oakleaf lettuce

Wash and grate the courgettes without peeling them. Wash and coarsely chop the spring onions. Boil a saucepan of water and cook the pasta until it is *al dente* (just tender). Drain and return to the pan. Add the olive oil and lemon juice, the courgettes, chopped spring onions, mangetout peas, and baby sweetcorn. Toss, turn into a dish lined with oakleaf lettuce leaves, sprinkle with the chopped parsley, and serve at once.

Pasta shells with broccoli serves 4

375g (12oz) fresh broccoli
4tbs olive oil
squeeze of anchovy paste
generous pinch of chilli
    powder – or a deseeded,
    chopped-up, small chilli,
    according to preference
black pepper, freshly milled
375g (12oz) pasta shells or
    other pasta
a big nut of butter
3tbs Parmesan cheese, grated

Put plenty of water on to boil for the pasta. Wash the broccoli and break into small florets. Cook in boiling water until tender – 5–6 minutes. Drain. Heat the oil in a large frying pan, and add the anchovy paste and the chilli or chilli powder. Add the broccoli, sprinkle with pepper, and sauté for 5 minutes. Keep the sauce warm while you cook the pasta. When it's ready, drain, return to the saucepan, add the butter and cheese, and toss. Turn into a warmed dish, add the sauce, and fold in quickly.

Meatballs and tomato sauce serves 4

500g (1lb) minced beef
3 cloves garlic, chopped
1tbs chopped fresh mint
1tbs chopped fresh parsley
salt and black pepper
1 egg
2tbs olive oil
Tomato sauce (p.189)

This is an American-style recipe that turns spaghetti into a substantial meal.

Mix together the minced beef, garlic, fresh herbs, and salt and pepper. Break the egg into the mixture and mix it up with your hands. Form the mixture into meatballs the size of table-tennis balls. Heat the oil in a frying pan and fry the meatballs gently for 7–10 minutes. When they are cooked through, add them to the tomato sauce, and serve with spaghetti, cooked until it is just tender.

Big Macks serves 4

CIRCULATORY · FATIGUE · JOINTS · URINARY

250g (8oz) cooked mackerel
    or mackerel tinned in brine
175g (6oz) mashed potato
30g (1oz) butter
2-3 spring onions, cleaned
    and chopped
1tbs fresh parsley, chopped
1tbs milk
1tbs fine oatmeal
2tbs vegetable oil
watercress and tomatoes
    to garnish

Skin and bone the mackerel. Flake, and mix with the mashed potatoes and melted butter. Add the spring onions. If the mixture is very stiff, moisten with a little milk. Shape into burgers and chill for at least half an hour.

When you are ready to eat, dust the burgers with oatmeal and fry until golden brown on both sides. Drain on kitchen paper. Serve with watercress and slices of tomato. Big Macks can also be eaten cold, in a wholemeal bun or bap, with cress and slices of cucumber.

Haddock and broccoli au gratin serves 4

CIRCULATORY · DIGESTIVE · JOINTS · FATIGUE

500g (1lb) broccoli
30g (1oz) butter
30g (1oz) plain white flour
450ml (¾pt) milk
125g (4oz) grated Cheddar
salt and pepper
750g (1½lb) haddock fillets,
    skinned

Steam the broccoli until barely tender. Melt the butter and stir in the flour. Add the milk, heated to near boiling point, stir, and bring to the boil. Add half the cheese, and a little salt and pepper. Butter an ovenproof casserole dish, put in the broccoli, lay the haddock fillets on top, and pour over the cheese sauce. Sprinkle with the rest of the cheese. Heat the oven to 180°C (350°F/gas 4), for 30-40 minutes, when the top should be golden and bubbling.

Grilled garlicky gambas serves 4

CANCER · CIRCULATORY · STRESS · RESPIRATORY · SKIN

16 20 big Pacific prawns in their shells (fresh are best, but if you do use frozen, thaw them thoroughly and blot completely dry)
3-4 large cloves garlic
2tbs olive oil
lettuce leaves for garnish
chunks of lemon for serving

Wash and dry the prawns if fresh. Chop the garlic up very small, put in a small bowl, and add the olive oil. Marinate for a couple of hours. Turn the grill on high, use a pastry brush to paint the prawns with the garlicky oil, and grill until the shells are almost burned. Serve on a bed of lettuce, with chunks of lemon to squeeze over them.

Salmon with green sauce serves 2

CANCER · CIRCULATORY · RESPIRATORY

2 150g (5oz) fresh salmon steaks
½ thick slice of wholewheat bread with crusts removed
2tbs lemon juice
1 clove garlic, finely chopped
2tbs pine nuts
2tbs fresh parsley, finely chopped
2tbs fresh basil, finely chopped (if no basil, use all parsley)
yolk of 1 hard-boiled egg, mashed
175ml (6fl oz) extra-virgin olive oil
a sprig of fresh parsley to garnish

To make the sauce: soak the bread in the lemon juice for 10 minutes. Mash it up in a mixing bowl. Add the garlic, pine nuts, parsley, basil, and mashed egg yolk. Combine and mash with a fork. Dribble in the oil a little at a time, beating as you do so. Leave to stand for at least an hour before you need it, so that the flavours can mingle. (You can also make the sauce in a blender or food processor: put in the ingredients except the oil, blend them together very lightly, then add the oil first in a trickle and then in a steady stream with the blades running.) When you're ready to eat, brush the steaks with a little olive oil on each side and heat under a red-hot grill until just forming a crust on each side and turning brown at the edges. Serve on hot plates and spoon the sauce around, but not over, the steaks. Garnish with parsley, and serve with boiled new potatoes.

Sardines with mustard sauce serves 4

CANCER · CIRCULATORY · STRESS · JOINTS · SKIN

12–16 sardines
1 tbs olive oil
150g (5oz) low-fat natural
  yoghurt
1 tbs fresh parsley, finely
chopped
1 tbs Dijon mustard
1 lemon, quartered

Split and clean the sardines, brush with the oil, and grill under a red-hot grill for a minute or so on either side. Combine the yoghurt, parsley, and mustard to make the sauce. Serve the sardines with this sauce, and a quarter of the lemon for each serving.

Herb-coated sea bass serves 4

CANCER · FATIGUE · RESPIRATORY · SKIN · URINARY

2 medium-sized onions,
  finely chopped
1 tbs mixed fennel, parsley,
  and tarragon, chopped
150ml (¼pt) water and dry
  white wine (mixed half
  and half)
1 1kg (2lb) sea-bass, washed
  and dried
1 tbs olive oil
1 lemon
30g (1oz) butter
salt and pepper

Combine the onion and herbs with the water and wine. Slice the lemon thinly and remove the seeds. Lay the cleaned and dried fish in an oval, ovenproof baking dish and moisten with the olive oil. Pour the wine-and-herb mixture over it, cover with the slices of lemon, dot with the butter and season to taste. Bake in the oven at 230°C (450°F/gas 8) for 25–30 minutes. Baste while cooking.

Herrings in oatmeal serves 4

CIRCULATORY · STRESS · JOINTS · SKIN

4 fresh herrings (ask your
  fishmonger to split and
  trim them)
60g (2oz) coarse oatmeal
freshly ground black pepper
2tbs sunflower or
  grapeseed oil
1 lemon, quartered
2tbs fresh parsley, chopped

Wash and pat dry the herrings and put the
oatmeal on a plate with a generous sprinkling of
freshly ground black pepper. Dip the herrings in
the oatmeal and turn them over until completely
coated. Heat the oil to smoking point in a large
frying pan and fry the herrings until golden
brown – 3-4 minutes each side. Serve them
immediately with a wedge of lemon and a
sprinkle of parsley.

Prawn, broccoli, and leek stir-fry serves 2

CANCER · CIRCULATORY

2tbs sunflower oil
1 clove garlic, crushed
125g (4oz) broccoli florets
1 leek, finely sliced
1tbs dark soy sauce
4tbs vegetable stock (p.188)
1 tomato, chopped
1tbs plain flour
125g (4oz) cooked prawns
1 carrot, peeled and cut into
  thin matchsticks
2.5cm (1in) piece fresh
  ginger, cut into thin
  matchsticks
90g (3oz) fresh watercress
Any green vegetable can be
  used in this recipe

Heat the oil in a large frying pan or wok and
quickly fry, but do not brown, the garlic. Add
the broccoli, and cook for 2 minutes, then add
the leek, and cook for another minute, stirring
constantly. Stir in the soy sauce, stock, and
tomato. Mix the flour with 2 tablespoons of water
to make a smooth paste, and stir into the sauce.
Cook until thickened. Add the prawns, carrot,
and ginger, and cook over a rapid heat for
1 minute. Stir in the watercress, and serve
immediately.

Peppered fish with vinaigrette serves 4 ▶

CIRCULATORY · DIGESTIVE · RESPIRATORY

1 heaped tbs mixed
   peppercorns
1 heaped tbs plain flour,
   seasoned with a little salt
2 fresh or frozen white fish
   fillets, each weighing
   approx. 200g (7oz)
1 tbs olive oil

For the vinaigrette:
1 clove garlic, crushed
2 tsp coarse-grain mustard
grated rind and juice of
   2 limes
4 tbs olive oil
salt and freshly ground black
   pepper
fresh coriander, chopped

This delicious recipe was presented in a leaflet by a British supermarket to their customers.

Coarsely crush the peppercorns and mix them together with the seasoned flour. Skin the fish fillets, wipe with kitchen paper, and coat them with the peppercorn mixture, pressing it well onto both sides. Set aside. Meanwhile, prepare the vinaigrette. Combine in a bowl the garlic, mustard, lime rind and juice, 4 tablespoons of oil, salt, pepper, and coriander.

Heat a tablespoon of olive oil in a large frying pan. When hot, add the fish and fry for 3 minutes on each side, until crisp and golden. Keeping the heat high, pour the vinaigrette around the fish, and maintain heat for a couple of minutes to reduce the liquid.

Baked fish provençal serves 2

DIGESTIVE · FATIGUE · RESPIRATORY

750g (1½lb) skinned white
   fish
2 tbs dry white wine
juice of 1 lemon
1 tbs oil
1 medium-sized onion
2 cloves garlic
1 425g (14oz) tin of tomatoes,
   roughly chopped
mixed herbs, salt, and pepper
1 tbs fresh parsley, chopped

Put the fish into a shallow casserole dish, and pour over the white wine and lemon juice. Leave to marinate. Chop the onion and garlic finely, heat the oil, and cook them until soft. Remove the fish from its marinade, drain, and add the marinade to the onion and garlic. Let it reduce a little, then add the tomatoes and herbs and season. Wipe and lightly oil the casserole, put in the fish fillets, pour over the sauce, and bake at 200°C (400°F/gas 6) for 20 minutes. Sprinkle with parsley and serve.

Prawn and tomato curry serves 4 ▶

CANCER · CIRCULATORY

1 medium-sized onion, chopped
425g (14oz) tin of tomatoes
1 clove garlic, chopped
2tbs fresh coriander, chopped
3tbs frozen peas
½ vegetable stock cube
1tsp ground cumin
1tsp ground coriander
a good squeeze of tomato
   paste from a tube
salt
1tsp Garam Masala
2tbs curry powder
1 red chilli, deseeded and
   chopped
375g (12oz) prawns, shelled
   and cooked (if using frozen,
   defrost in the fridge all day)
150ml (¼pt) single cream

Put the onion, tomatoes with their juice, garlic, half of the fresh coriander, frozen peas, and crumbled stock cube in a pan. Let them simmer for about 5 minutes.

Make a paste with the cumin, ground coriander, tomato paste, salt, and a little water. Add the Garam Masala, curry powder, and chilli. Add this mixture to the tomato sauce, and simmer for about 5 minutes.

Add the prawns, and let them simmer in the sauce for a further 3 minutes – no longer or they will go leathery. Then turn off the heat, stir in the cream, sprinkle with the rest of the fresh coriander, and serve at once with plain boiled rice. To make this a more substantial dish, add a tin of sweetcorn in unsweetened water to the tomato sauce.

Cod with sesame and spinach serves 2

CANCER · CIRCULATORY · DIGESTIVE · FATIGUE · URINARY

2 white fish steaks
salt and pepper
1 egg, beaten
60g (2oz) sesame seeds
a knob of butter
250g (8oz) young spinach
¼tsp nutmeg, freshly grated
2tbs crème fraîche

Heat the oven to 175°C (350°F/gas 4). Season the fish with salt and pepper, brush with beaten egg, and coat the fish with sesame seeds. Place the fish on a baking sheet and cook in the oven for 20 minutes. Just before serving, melt the butter in a large frying pan and wilt the spinach leaves in it. Add the nutmeg, salt and pepper to taste, and the crème fraîche. Divide between two plates, resting the cod on top. Serve with lemon wedges.

Hearty beef stew serves 4

STRESS · FATIGUE · RESPIRATORY

1 large onion
1 tbs olive oil
2 cloves garlic
500g (1lb) lean rump steak,
    cubed
2 heaped tbs wholewheat
    flour, well seasoned
150ml (¼pt) red wine
600ml (1pt) vegetable stock
    (*p.188*)
2 large carrots, sliced
1 large leek, cut into chunks
1 stick celery, thickly sliced
1 parsnip, thickly sliced
1 bay leaf
6 peppercorns
a sprig of fresh thyme

Cut the onion in half, finely chop one half, and slice the other. Heat the oil in a heavy-bottomed pan and soften the chopped onion and the garlic. Then toss the cubes of meat in the flour so that each cube is liberally covered. Add the floured meat to the pan and stir briskly over a high heat to sear all the surfaces. Reduce the heat, add the wine, bring to the boil, and let it bubble for a couple of minutes. Then add the stock and all the vegetables and seasonings. Cover the pan tightly, turn the heat down, and simmer, stirring occasionally, for about an hour and a half. Add more stock or boiling water if it looks dry.

Carpaccio serves 4

FATIGUE · RESPIRATORY

300g (10oz) best fillet steak
    (get your butcher to slice it
    paper-thin for you, or
    sharpen your best knife
    and do it yourself!)
1 small bunch rocket or
    watercress
1 bunch celery leaves
4 tbs Parmesan cheese,
    freshly grated
4 tsp extra-virgin olive oil
freshly ground black pepper

Pound the slices of steak between 2 sheets of waxed paper until they are as thin as possible. Arrange on individual plates and decorate with the rocket or watercress and celery leaves. Sprinkle over the Parmesan, drizzle over 1 teaspoon of oil per steak, and add a generous amount of freshly ground black pepper. Serve with coarse wholemeal bread.

NOTE: The recipe requires the very finest and freshest of ingredients. Tough steak, stale Parmesan, or poor-quality oil could ruin it.

Italian pan-fried liver serves 2

STRESS · FATIGUE

3tbs sunflower oil
30g (1oz) butter
1 onion, coarsely chopped
2 rashers bacon, stretched
    with the back of a knife,
    and cut in two
375g (12oz) calf's liver, thinly
    sliced
salt and pepper
3tbs fino, or other dry sherry
a handful of chopped parsley

The last minute addition of dry sherry makes a delicious sauce, but if no sherry is to be found, use vermouth, or failing that, just water.

Heat the oil and butter together until foaming, and then add the onion. Cook until softened and beginning to brown. Remove the onion, and add the bacon. Cook until just beginning to brown, then remove. Season the liver with salt and pepper, and sauté it over a high heat for 1 minute on either side, or until it is just turning brown. Return the onions and bacon to the pan, and pour in the sherry. Heat until bubbling, and a sauce has formed. Stir in the parsley, and serve immediately.

Lamb and pine nut koftas serves 4

FATIGUE

1 onion
60g (2oz) pine nuts
500g (1lb) minced lamb
1tbs fresh mint, chopped
1 egg, beaten

Heat the grill to maximum. Place the onion and pine nuts in a food processor and chop finely. Add the lamb, mint, and egg, and blend to a smooth paste. Shape into walnut-sized balls or small sausage shapes and press tightly onto kebab sticks. Grill for 2 minutes on each side. Serve with wholewheat pitta bread, lemon wedges, and a green salad of rocket, watercress, and cos.

Lamb burgers serves 4 ▶

STRESS · FATIGUE · RESPIRATORY

1 slice wholemeal bread
  with crusts removed
500g (1lb) minced lamb
1 large onion, finely chopped
1 egg
a good pinch of dried oregano
a good pinch of dried thyme
1tbs fresh parsley, chopped
1tbs fresh mint, chopped
salt and freshly ground black
  pepper

Soak the bread in water, then squeeze out the excess. If you have a food processor you can put in all the other ingredients and process them briefly – chop the onion finely first. However, it's quite easy to mix them by hand. Crumble the bread into a bowl with the minced lamb. Some supermarkets sell low-fat, ready-minced lamb, or you can buy fillets, and mince them in a food processor. Add the onion. Beat the egg, and add it. Add the herbs, salt and pepper, and mix. This mixture can be left to gather flavour for 2–3 hours, or you can leave it all day in the refrigerator in a bowl covered with cling film.

When you're ready to cook, heat the grill to maximum, shape the lamb mixture into burgers, oil the grill rack, and grill for 3–4 minutes on each side. Serve with Tomato sauce (*p.189*).

Ginger lamb stir-fry serves 4

STRESS · FATIGUE · RESPIRATORY

375g (12oz) lean lamb
2tsp dry sherry
4tsp soy sauce
½tsp sesame oil
2tsp olive oil
white part of 1 leek, sliced
1 spring onion, chopped
2 cloves garlic, thinly sliced
2.5cm (1in) piece of fresh
  ginger, peeled and grated

Remove all fat from the lamb and cut it into thick strips. Put it in a flat dish with the sherry, soy sauce, and sesame oil, and leave to marinate for 30 minutes. Drain, reserving the marinade. Heat a wok or frying pan and add the olive oil, then the lamb with some marinade. Stir for 3 minutes over a high heat. Add the leeks and stir for 2 minutes, then add the spring onions, garlic, and ginger, and stir for another 3 minutes.

Devilled chicken serves 4

CIRCULATORY · DIGESTIVE · FATIGUE · RESPIRATORY

8 chicken drumsticks – allow
  2 per person
2 cloves garlic, crushed
5tbs Dijon mustard
2tbs olive oil
2tsp cayenne pepper
5cm (2in) fresh ginger,
  peeled and grated
1tsp soft brown sugar
a dash or two of
  Worcestershire sauce
salt and pepper

Tangy spices, such as mustard and chilli, are often assumed to be deadly to the disordered digestive system. In fact, unless you consume them in heroic quantities, they can actually be beneficial to the gut, toning and stimulating the digestive action. Mustard is one such spice. We found this recipe (originally for Devilled Turkey) in a splendid book devoted to a herb that has been cultivated since at least 4000bc, and is the second most common condiment in the world. *The Compleat Mustard* is by Rosemary Man and Robin Weir.

Score the drumsticks deeply in several places, then mix the garlic with the mustard, oil, cayenne, grated ginger, sugar, and Worcestershire sauce. Season lightly with salt and pepper and paint each drumstick, liberally and evenly, with the paste. Chill for a minimum of 12 hours, bringing to room temperature before cooking.

Heat the grill to very hot, then turn it low and cook the drumsticks for 30–40 minutes. Turn frequently and baste with any juices that have poured off them until they are very dark and the meat is cooked through. Then turn the grill to high and cook for 3–4 minutes, turning them round to warm thoroughly and crisp up the skin. Serve hot or cold, with a sharp green salad.

If you use turkey drumsticks, allow one for each person, and extend the cooking time to around 1½ hours.

Spicy chicken wings — serves 4

CIRCULATORY · DIGESTIVE · RESPIRATORY

750g (1½lb) chicken wings,
   with the tips removed
8tbs tomato ketchup
3tbs Worcestershire sauce
1tbs runny honey
3tsp paprika
3tsp English dried mustard
   powder
1tsp turmeric
salt and freshly ground
   black pepper

Put the chicken in a flat dish. Combine the other ingredients and pour over the chicken, reserving a few tablespoons. Leave to marinate for 15 minutes, turning the chicken a few times.

Heat the grill and line the grill pan with foil. Cook the chicken for 10–12 minutes, turning them 2–3 times and basting them with the remaining marinade. Serve with a large salad – and plenty of paper napkins, as the only way to eat these is with your fingers – and a cold beer.

Chicken with garlic — serves 4

CIRCULATORY · STRESS · RESPIRATORY

3tbs extra-virgin olive oil
15g (½oz) butter
4 leg quarters of chicken
salt and plenty of freshly
   ground black pepper
at least 10 large cloves garlic
   – up to 30 if you're brave!
300ml (½pt) dry white wine
1tbs fresh parsley, chopped

This recipe is good for the heart, but is not for the faint-hearted! Heat the oil and butter in a large, deep frying pan. Season the chicken with salt and pepper, add it to the pan, and cook until it is evenly browned on both sides for 8–10 minutes. Reduce the heat, and place the unpeeled cloves of garlic under the chicken on the bottom of the pan. Cook for a further 10 minutes, shaking the pan regularly, then add the wine, and scrape all the cooking bits from around the pan with a wooden spoon. Continue cooking for another 8–10 minutes until the chicken is thoroughly cooked.

Arrange the golden garlic around the pieces of chicken, and sprinkle with the parsley. Serve with bread and the rest of the dry white wine.

Chicken livers with warm salad

CIRCULATORY · RESPIRATORY · SKIN

750g (1½lb) chicken livers –
    preferably free-range
4tbs walnut oil
1½tbs red wine vinegar
4 cloves garlic, finely chopped
pepper and salt
1 small head radicchio
1 bunch watercress
1 head chicory
50g (2oz) butter

Wash the livers and pat dry. Put 4 plates to warm in the oven until very hot. Make the salad dressing with the oil, vinegar, finely-chopped garlic, pepper, and salt. Wash and dry the salad leaves, pulling the radicchio apart and separating the watercress into sprigs and the chicory into its long leaves. Melt the butter in a heavy non-stick frying pan, toss the livers for about 5 minutes, then remove the pan from the heat. Quickly arrange the radicchio, watercress, and chicory leaves on the 4 hot plates. Remove the livers from the pan with a slotted spoon and distribute among the plates. Pour the dressing over and serve at once. (Have an oven-cloth handy and warn diners that the plates are hot!)

Bedouin chicken serves 4 ▶

CIRCULATORY · FATIGUE · RESPIRATORY · URINARY

1tsp oil
1 small onion, finely chopped
60g (2oz) cooked barley (*p.189*)
1 small apple, diced
4 fresh dates, stoned and
    chopped
30g (1oz) raisins, well washed
1tsp chopped almonds
½tsp allspice
½tsp cinnamon
1 1.4kg (3lb) chicken
salt and pepper
juice of half a lemon
1 lemon, quartered to garnish

Heat the oil and fry the onion until just transparent. Put it, together with all the other stuffing ingredients and spices, in a mixing bowl, and combine. Stuff the chicken with the mixture, tie it up, put it in a roasting pan, and season liberally with pepper, salt, and a squeeze of lemon juice. Heat the oven to 220°C (425°F/gas 7.) Put in the chicken and cook for 10 minutes, then turn the oven down to 190°C (375°F/gas 5), and roast for 1¼ hours or until the juices run clear from the thigh when you pierce it with a skewer

Eat with a plain lettuce salad and a lemon and oil dressing.

Sun-dried tomato risotto serves 4

CANCER · CIRCULATORY · FATIGUE

2tbs vegetable oil
1 medium-sized onion,
    chopped
2 cloves garlic, chopped
250g (8oz) brown rice
175g (6oz) sun-dried
    tomatoes, chopped
750ml (1¼pt) vegetable stock
    (p.188)
4 ripe red tomatoes, peeled
    and chopped
salt and freshly ground black
    pepper
1tbs fresh basil, chopped
2tbs grated Cheddar,
    Parmesan, or other
    hard cheese

Heat the oil, and fry the onion and garlic for 2–3 minutes. Add the rice, sun-dried tomatoes – drain them first if they are in oil – stock, and fresh tomatoes. Bring to the boil, season with salt and pepper to taste, and simmer for approximately 40 minutes. Add the basil, and stir in the cheese before serving.

NOTE: For a quicker version of this recipe, you can use boil-in-the-bag or easy-cook brown rice. While it's cooking according to the packet's instructions, heat the oil, and fry the onion and garlic until they are just changing colour. Add the sun-dried and fresh tomatoes, and sauté for another 5 minutes. When the rice is ready, stir it into the tomato mixture, season to taste, add the basil, stir in the cheese, and serve.

Red hot rice serves 4

CIRCULATORY · DIGESTIVE · FATIGUE · RESPIRATORY

125g (4oz) boil-in-the-bag
    brown rice
1 small red pepper
1 small, fresh red chilli
3tbs vegetable oil
1 medium-sized onion,
    finely sliced
2 cloves garlic, finely sliced

Boil a pan of water, and cook the rice – it will take 20–25 minutes. Meanwhile, wash the pepper, remove the ribs and seeds, and slice it into strips. Wash, slit open, and deseed the chilli – rinse your hands carefully afterwards. Heat the oil, and gently sauté the chilli in it for 5 minutes, then fish it out with a fork, and discard it. Add the onion, garlic, and red pepper, and sauté them over a low heat until they are soft. When the rice is cooked, put it in a salad bowl, pour in the contents of the frying pan, and stir through.

Bean casserole serves 4

CANCER · CIRCULATORY · JOINTS · RESPIRATORY · URINARY

60g (2oz) dried butter beans, soaked overnight
60g (2oz) dried red kidney beans, soaked overnight
1 tbs vegetable oil
1 large onion, finely chopped
2 cloves garlic, finely chopped
2 large carrots, sliced
2 courgettes, sliced
2 sticks celery, sliced
200g (7oz) tinned tomatoes
a small sprig of fresh thyme or a pinch of dried thyme
salt and pepper

Drain the beans, put in separate pans, and cover with cold water. Bring to the boil and boil rapidly for 10 minutes, then turn the heat down, cover, and simmer for about an hour, or until the beans are tender. Drain, reserving the liquid. Heat the oil in a heavy pan, add the onion and garlic, and let them soften. Add the carrots, courgettes, celery, tomatoes, thyme, and salt and pepper to taste. Add enough of the bean cooking water to moisten. Cover and simmer for about 15 minutes, adding more of the bean water if necessary, until all the vegetables are soft. Add the beans – and more liquid as needed – cover, heat through gently, and serve.

Quick bean ragout serves 4

CANCER · CIRCULATORY · DIGESTIVE · SKIN

1 tbs olive oil
1 tsp dill seeds
4 cloves garlic, finely chopped
1 small onion, finely chopped
1 Savoy cabbage, shredded
600ml (1pt) vegetable stock (p.188)
60g (2oz) each tinned flageolet beans, kidney beans, black beans, and soybeans
250g (8oz) each tinned borlotti beans, fresh runner beans, and shelled broad beans
1 tbs fresh parsley, chopped

A seven-bean sampling for real bean addicts – using tinned beans, without all that pre-soaking.

Heat the oil in a big casserole. Sweat the dill seeds, garlic, and onion until soft. Add the shredded cabbage and stir briskly. Add the stock. Open all the tins of beans and rinse them under running cold water (you can use up the surplus in a salad). Add them, bring to the boil and simmer for 20 minutes. Then add the broad beans and the runner beans. Cook for another 10 minutes. Serve sprinkled with the parsley.

Vegetable risotto serves 4 ▶

CANCER · CIRCULATORY · STRESS · JOINTS · RESPIRATORY

3tbs olive oil
2 cloves garlic, chopped
2 large onions, sliced
125g (4oz) whole unsalted
    peanuts
2 sticks celery, sliced
2 large carrots, sliced
1 large leek, sliced
375g (12oz) brown rice,
    washed
900ml (1½pt) vegetable stock
    (*p.188*)
125g (4oz) button mushrooms
salt and pepper
125g (4oz) cucumber, peeled
    and diced

Heat the oil in a large frying pan or skillet, and sauté the garlic, onions, and peanuts. Add the celery, carrot, and leek, and sauté for another 5 minutes, stirring frequently. Add the rice and continue to stir for another 5 minutes. Add the stock, mushrooms, and salt and pepper to taste, and bring to the boil. After 6-7 minutes, add the cucumber. Cover and simmer until the rice is tender and all the liquid is absorbed. Add more stock to the mixture if necessary.

Warm bulgur with aubergines serves 4

CIRCULATORY · STRESS · FATIGUE

125g (4oz) bulgur or cracked
    wheat
4-6tbs olive oil
1 large onion, thinly sliced
1 large aubergine, cut into
    cubes
2tsp ground coriander
2tsp ground cumin
90g (3oz) flaked almonds
60g (2oz) raisins
salt and freshly ground black
    pepper

Simmer the bulgur wheat in twice its volume of water for 10 minutes, or until the grains are soft. Drain if necessary. Meanwhile, heat a little oil and fry the onion until it turns brown. Add the aubergine and, stirring frequently, sauté until it is brown – you might need to add a little extra oil. Add the coriander and cumin to the pan and cook for 1 minute, stirring constantly. Lower the heat, add the almonds and raisins, and brown lightly. Stir the cooked bulgur wheat into the vegetables, season with salt and pepper, add extra oil, and sauté for 1 minute to heat through.

Rainbow peppers serves 4

CANCER · CIRCULATORY · DIGESTIVE · FATIGUE · JOINTS

90g (3oz) brown rice
150ml (¼pt) vegetable stock
   (*p.188*)
1tsp salt, plus extra to taste
   for seasoning
2tbs olive oil
1 large onion, chopped
2 cloves garlic, chopped
1tbs currants
1tbs pine nuts
juice of 1 lemon
1 tbs oregano
freshly ground black pepper
4 peppers: 1 red,
   1 yellow, 1 green, and
   1 orange
1tbs tomato purée
150ml (¼pt) water

An hour before you want to start preparing the dish, cook the rice. Wash it thoroughly and put it in a small ovenproof casserole. Add 1 teaspoon of salt and enough stock to come up to the depth of a thumbnail over the surface of the rice. Cover tightly, and cook in an oven pre-heated to 175°C (350°F/gas 4). After 35–40 minutes, the rice should have absorbed all the stock and be cooked through but still slightly moist.

Heat 1 tablespoon of the oil, and soften the onions in it. Add the chopped garlic, and cook for a moment longer. Add the onion and garlic to the cooked rice, together with the currants, pine nuts, lemon juice, oregano, a little freshly ground pepper, and a touch of salt to taste.

Wash the peppers, then slice the tops off and reserve them. Scrape out the seeds and fibrous ribs, pack with the rice mixture, and replace the tops. Stand the peppers in an oven-dish just big enough to hold them, so that they don't collapse sideways; if necessary, slice off a sliver from the bottoms to steady them. Brush with oil and stir the tomato purée into the water and pour it in. Place in an oven pre-heated to 200°C (400°F/gas 6). Bake for about 45 minutes, checking periodically to ensure the liquid hasn't dried out, adding a little more water or stock if necessary.

Serve with Tomato sauce (*p.189*) and a green vegetable or a salad.

Braised red cabbage serves 4

CIRCULATORY · FATIGUE

1 medium-sized red cabbage
3tbs olive oil
1 large onion, chopped
3 garlic cloves, chopped
4–5tbs apple cider vinegar
1tsp brown sugar
salt and pepper

Rinse the cabbage, shred and drain. Heat the oil, sauté the onion gently, add the garlic and cabbage, and stir until well mixed. Add the vinegar and sugar, and salt and pepper to taste. Lower the heat and cook covered, stirring occasionally, until tender – about half an hour – or cook covered in a moderate oven. If you like, add a dash of lemon before serving.

Tofu and vegetable stir-fry serves 4

CIRCULATORY · FATIGUE · JOINTS · SKIN · URINARY

3tbs vegetable oil
250g (8oz) tofu
1 medium-sized onion, finely
   chopped
1 green pepper, chopped
1tsp grated fresh ginger
1 stick celery, chopped
2 medium-sized carrots, sliced
a chunk of cabbage, cut into
   thin wedges
4–5 mushrooms, sliced
125g (4oz) cashews
250ml (8fl oz) vegetable stock
   (*p.188*)
a dash of soy sauce

Heat the oil in the wok, add the tofu, and fry lightly until golden brown. Remove with a slotted spoon and leave on one side. Sauté the onion, green pepper, ginger, and celery over medium heat until soft but not brown. Add the carrots and the cabbage and sauté for 3–4 minutes; then add the mushrooms and cashews and sauté for 1 minute more. Add a cup of stock, return the tofu, cover, and steam until the vegetables are soft. Stir in a dash of soy sauce.

Cabbage with onion and bacon serves 4

CIRCULATORY · FATIGUE

1 medium-sized cabbage
1tbs vegetable oil
1 medium-sized onion,
   coarsely chopped
3-4 rashers streaky bacon,
   cut in pieces
salt and pepper

Wash and shred the cabbage, but don't dry it. Heat the oil in a big saucepan, and gently fry the onion and bacon together until the onion is just changing colour, and the bacon is nearly crisp. Add the cabbage, salt and pepper, and stir. Put the lid on, turn down the heat, and simmer. Shake the pan, and give the contents a stir a couple of times – the cabbage will steam cook – until the cabbage is cooked *al dente* (just tender).

Spiced red cabbage serves 4

CIRCULATORY · FATIGUE

1 small red cabbage
1 large cooking apple, peeled
   and sliced in segments
3tbs red wine vinegar
10 cloves
salt and pepper
1-2tsp brown sugar

Wash and shred the cabbage and put it in a pan with the apple, red wine vinegar, cloves, and salt and pepper. Sprinkle over 2-3 tablespoons of water, add the brown sugar, cover, and simmer for 20 minutes.

Potato galette serves 4

CIRCULATORY · DIGESTIVE · FATIGUE

4 medium-sized potatoes
2 egg yolks
1 medium-sized onion, grated
3tbs fresh parsley, chopped
2 cloves garlic, finely chopped
1tsp plain flour
1tsp ground nutmeg
sunflower or corn oil

Peel the potatoes and grate in a food processor. Turn into a bowl and mix with the egg yolks, onion, parsley, and garlic. Form into a cake and dust with flour. Heat enough oil in a frying pan to come about half way up the side of the cake. Add the cake and fry on both sides until golden. Drain on kitchen paper and dust with nutmeg.

Ratatouille serves 4

CANCER · CIRCULATORY · DIGESTIVE · URINARY

2 courgettes
1 large aubergine
salt
2 large red peppers
1 large onion
2 cloves garlic
4tbs extra-virgin olive oil
1 small tin of tomatoes
a few coriander seeds or ½tsp
    ground coriander
1tbs fresh basil or parsley,
    chopped

Wash the courgettes and aubergine and cut into small slices. Place in a colander, sprinkle with salt, and leave for an hour.

Deseed the peppers and cut into thin strips. Peel and finely slice the onion and garlic. Heat the oil in a heavy-bottomed saucepan. Add the onion and sweat until transparent. Rinse and pat dry the aubergines and courgettes, and add them, together with the peppers and garlic. Cover and simmer gently for about 40 minutes. Add the tomatoes and coriander, and cook for another 30 minutes – but don't let it get too mushy. Stir in the basil or parsley, and serve hot.

Grilled red radicchio serves 4

CANCER · CIRCULATORY · DIGESTIVE · JOINTS

2–3 radicchio heads
3–4tbs extra-virgin olive oil
salt and freshly ground
    pepper
lemon slices

Clean the radicchio, stripping off wilted outer leaves. Slice thickly, rinse, and pat completely dry with kitchen paper. Lay the slices in a shallow, ovenproof dish. Mix 3–4 tablespoons of oil with a little salt and freshly ground pepper, and pour over the radicchio. Leave it to soften for 5 minutes, while you heat the grill. Grill for no longer than it takes for the leaves to change colour a little. Lift out and serve with slices of lemon, and bread to mop up the tangy juices.

Cauliflower and broccoli cheese serves 4

CANCER · STRESS · FATIGUE

1 small cauliflower
1 small head of broccoli
500ml (16fl oz) milk
60g (2oz) butter
1 tbs wholemeal flour
60g (2oz) Cheddar, grated
1 tsp Dijon mustard
salt and pepper

Preheat the oven to 180°C (350°F/gas 1). Break the vegetables into florets and cook them in the milk until just tender. Drain, reserving the milk, and put the vegetables in a buttered gratin dish. Melt the butter in a saucepan. Stir in the flour, 1 tablespoon of the cheese, the mustard, and seasoning. Stir in the hot milk to make a smooth sauce. Pour over the vegetables, scatter the rest of the cheese on top, and bake for 15–20 minutes.

Vegetable couscous serves 4

CANCER · DIGESTIVE · FATIGUE

olive oil, for frying
1 small onion, finely chopped
2 carrots, halved lengthways
    and sliced
1 courgette, halved
    lengthways and sliced
half red pepper, deseeded
    and chopped
1 tsp (or more to taste)
    ground cumin
3 tomatoes, skinned and diced
salt
1–2 tbs fresh coriander
    leaves
400g (13oz) tinned chickpeas,
    drained
150g (5oz) couscous

Heat a little olive oil in a frying pan. Add the onion and fry until golden. Add the carrots, courgette, red pepper, and ground cumin and continue to fry for a few minutes. Add the tomatoes, a little salt, and the coriander leaves. Simmer for about 10 minutes, or until the vegetables are cooked and nicely tender. Add the chickpeas and heat through. While the vegetables are cooking, steam the couscous, according to packet instructions. Serve the vegetables and steamed couscous together. If a child insists on having meat with this, you can fry a few small pieces of chicken with the onion.

Roasted vegetables serves 4 ▶

CANCER · CIRCULATORY · RESPIRATORY

1 red pepper, cored, deseeded,
    and cut into chunks
1 yellow pepper, cored,
    deseeded, and cut into
    chunks
2 onions, quartered
2 medium-sized or 4 small
    courgettes, thickly sliced
8 cherry tomatoes
4 cloves garlic, crushed
4tbs olive oil
salt and black pepper
1 bunch fresh coriander,
    basil, or parsley, chopped

Preheat the oven to 200°C (400°F/gas 6). Arrange all the vegetables and the garlic in a shallow roasting tin. Add the olive oil, and push the vegetables around until they are well coated with the oil. Sprinkle with a little salt and pepper, and roast in the oven for about 40 minutes, stirring once or twice. The vegetables should be tender and just starting to turn golden-brown. Sprinkle with the chopped fresh herbs.

Serve these vegetables with plain brown rice, couscous, or bulgur for an appetizing and colourful supper. The vegetables are also a delicious accompaniment to the Sunday roast, grilled fish or meat, or to a simple omelette.

Aromatic mushrooms serves 4

CIRCULATORY · DIGESTION · SKIN

500g (1lb) small white or flat
    field mushrooms
3tbs olive oil
2 cloves garlic, sliced in half
1 bay leaf
6-8 coriander seeds
salt and freshly ground
    black pepper

Clean the mushrooms, and slice them thinly. Warm the olive oil in a pan. Add the garlic slices, bay leaf, coriander seeds, and salt and pepper. Add the mushrooms, and cover the pan. Shake gently, and cook over a very low heat for 20 minutes. Remove the bay leaf before serving the mushrooms.

Vegetable samosas serves 4

CIRCULATORY · DIGESTIVE

2 potatoes, cut into cubes

125g (4oz) finely chopped
   vegetables – use
   combinations of favourite
   vegetables, such as carrots,
   beans, peas, spinach,
   cauliflower, and parsnips

1tsp mild curry powder or
   paste

2tbs cream cheese or
   cottage cheese

salt and pepper

1tbs olive oil

30g (1oz) butter, melted

8 sheets filo pastry

4tbs poppy seeds or black
   sesame seeds

Preheat the oven to 190°C (375°F/gas 5). Boil the potato cubes in lightly salted water for about 10 minutes, or until soft. Drain well. In a separate pan, bring enough water to the boil to just cover the chopped vegetables and cook them until tender but still crisp. Drain well and put the vegetables and potatoes into a bowl. Add the curry powder or paste, cheese and salt and pepper. Mix everything really well together.

Melt the olive oil and butter in a small saucepan. Lay out one sheet of filo pastry and brush it with the melted butter and oil. Lay another sheet on top and brush again. Now cut the pastry lengthways into strips about 7cm (3in) wide. Put a heaped teaspoon of filling at one end of a strip. Fold the pastry diagonally across so that it makes a triangle. Keep folding over along the length of the strip until your triangle is completed. Brush the outside with butter and roll the samosa in poppy or black sesame seeds. Repeat with all your pastry and filling.

Put the samosas on a baking sheet and bake in the oven for 15–20 minutes, until golden. Serve the samosas while they are still warm. Makes about 16.

Sweet potato and nutmeg mash serves 4

DIGESTIVE · SKIN

2 large sweet potatoes,
   scrubbed and cubed
quarter head dark green
   cabbage, finely shredded
juice of a lemon
½tsp ground nutmeg
extra-virgin olive oil
freshly ground black pepper

This quick and easy recipe provides loads of slow release energy, betacarotene, and other essential carotenoids, together with protective vitamin C and anticancer chemicals from the cabbage and plenty of feel-good myristicine from the nutmeg. It's also rich in fibre. Serve as a side dish or top with an organic poached egg for a light supper or Sunday brunch.

Put the sweet potatoes in a large saucepan of cold water and bring to the boil uncovered. After 5 minutes, place the cabbage in a steamer on top and cover. Strain the sweet potatoes, put them back in the saucepan and on the heat, shaking vigorously until completely dry. Drizzle with olive oil, mash, stir in the steamed cabbage, add the nutmeg and pepper, and serve.

New potato and beer salad serves 4

CIRCULATORY · DIGESTIVE

1kg (2lb) new potatoes
1 red onion, finely chopped
2 cloves garlic, finely chopped
1tbs fresh thyme, chopped
1tbs flat-leaf parsley, chopped
6tbs extra-virgin olive oil
2tbs cider vinegar
175ml (6fl oz) beer
4 spring onions, chopped
1tbs wholegrain mustard
1tsp honey
pepper

Put the unpeeled potatoes in a large saucepan of cold water, bring to boil, and cook uncovered until just soft (about 20 minutes). Drain and leave until cool enough to handle. Cut each potato in half and mix gently with the onion, garlic, thyme, and parsley. To make the dressing, whisk all the other ingredients together to a smooth, creamy consistency. To serve, pour the dressing over the warm potatoes and serve immediately. If you're not going to eat this straight away, refrigerate the potatoes and dressing separately.

Tapenade serves 4

CIRCULATORY · JOINTS · RESPIRATORY

20 pitted black olives
1 tin anchovy fillets, drained
1 heaped tbs capers, rinsed
1tsp lemon juice
1 clove garlic
black pepper
100ml (3½fl oz) olive oil

Put all the ingredients except the oil in a blender and blend for a few seconds. Add black pepper to taste, and half a tablespoon of olive oil. Blend again and repeat, adding more oil until the mixture is a smooth, thick purée.

Falafel serves 4

CIRCULATORY · STRESS · JOINTS

250g (8oz) dried chickpeas
2 Spanish onions, finely
    chopped
3tbs fresh parsley,
    finely chopped
2tsp ground coriander
2tsp ground fennel
2tsp ground cumin
½tsp baking powder
4 cloves garlic, crushed
salt and freshly ground
    black pepper
2tbs flour (optional)
3-4tbs sunflower oil
paprika to garnish

Every cookery writer has their own version of falafel: our favourite is that of Paul Laurenson and Ethel Minogue published in *The Taste of Health* (BBC Books).

Soak the chickpeas in water for several hours until they double in size. Change the water as often as you remember during the soaking, as this reduces the likelihood of their causing flatulence. Blend the chickpeas with a little of their cooking water to a smooth paste. Add the onions and parsley to the chickpeas and blend again for a few seconds. Add all the ground spices, baking powder, crushed garlic, and salt and pepper. Knead the mixture for a moment or two to mix the ingredients well, then let it rest in the refrigerator for 30 minutes. Take small pieces and form into little flat cakes about 5cm (2in) across. If they are sticky, roll them in a little flour. Heat the oil and fry for about 2 minutes each side. Drain on kitchen paper, sprinkle with paprika, and serve hot or cold.

Pitta pizza serves 1

CANCER · FATIGUE

1 wholewheat pitta
1 medium-sized tomato, sliced
salt and freshly ground
    black pepper
a good pinch of dried oregano
1tbs Cheddar cheese, grated
1tsp olive oil

Made with wholewheat pitta bread, this is a superfast, healthy variation on pizza. Try any of the classic pizza toppings, such as anchovies, black olives, thinly sliced onion, slivers of red or green pepper, thin slices of mushroom, diced ham, or slices of pepperoni.

Heat the grill to red hot. Toast the pitta on one side for a minute or two, and remove from the grill. Turn the bread over, and top with sliced tomatoes, salt and pepper to taste, oregano, and the grated cheese. Dribble the oil over the top, and return to the grill. The pizza will be done in 2–3 minutes. This recipe serves one, but it can easily be multiplied to serve more.

Potato pancakes serves 4

CIRCULATORY · DIGESTIVE

500g (1lb) potatoes
1 medium-sized onion
2 eggs
2tbs plain flour
salt and pepper
3–4tbs sunflower oil

Peel the potatoes and onion, and grate them into a large bowl. Beat the eggs, and add them, stir in the flour and the salt and pepper. Mix together well. Heat the oil in a frying pan and fry tablespoonfuls of the mixture, flattening them down in the pan, for 5 minutes on each side.

Salade niçoise serves 4 ▶

CANCER · CIRCULATORY · STRESS · FATIGUE

1 head cos or iceberg
    lettuce
2 eggs
4 firm tomatoes
1 large red pepper
½ cucumber
4 small boiled potatoes
4 anchovy fillets
2tbs milk
2 cloves garlic, chopped
a pinch of mixed herbs
1½tbs good wine vinegar or
    balsamic vinegar
3tbs extra-virgin olive oil
12 pitted black olives

Wash and dry the lettuce. Hard boil and halve the eggs. Wash and quarter the tomatoes. Deseed the pepper and slice into strips. Peel and slice the cucumber. Halve the boiled potatoes. Soak the anchovy fillets for 30 minutes in the milk, then drain and dry.

Make the dressing by adding the garlic and mixed herbs to the vinegar and oil. Mix thoroughly, and leave to stand while you prepare the salad. Line the salad bowl with the lettuce leaves. Arrange all the other ingredients in the middle, decorate with the olives and anchovy fillets on top, and add the dressing just before you eat. Toss and serve.

Millet croquettes serves 4

CANCER · DIGESTIVE · STRESS

900ml (1½pt) water
300g (10oz) millet
4tbs oil
1 onion, finely chopped
2tbs parsley, freshly chopped
250g (8oz) grated cheese
salt and pepper
1 egg, beaten
1tbs wholemeal flour

Bring the water to the boil, add the millet, and simmer for about 25 minutes, stirring frequently, until the water is completely absorbed. In another pan, heat 2tbs of the oil, then melt the chopped onion. Add to the millet, together with the parsley and cheese, and season with salt and pepper to taste. Leave the mixture to cool. When cool, shape it into croquettes. Dip the croquettes in the beaten egg, then in the wholemeal flour, and fry in the rest of the oil until golden brown.

Banana and almond muffins serves 6

CIRCULATORY · DIGESTIVE · FATIGUE

175g (6oz) plain flour
1½tsp baking powder
1½tsp bicarbonate of soda
½tsp salt
2 eggs
6 large ripe bananas,
    thoroughly mashed
250g (8oz) dark brown sugar
90ml (2½fl oz) sunflower oil
90ml (2½fl oz) buttermilk
½tsp vanilla extract
100g (3½oz) almonds, toasted
    and chopped

Preheat the oven to 200°C (400°F/gas 6). Lightly grease a 12-cup muffin tin. Put the flour, baking powder, bicarbonate of soda, and salt in a large mixing bowl and mix well together. Mix the eggs, bananas, sugar, oil, buttermilk, and vanilla extract in a separate bowl and then pour them into the dry ingredients. Mix them together until just combined. (Be careful not to overmix or the muffins will be rubbery.) Fold in the almonds. Fill each muffin cup to the rim with batter. Bake for 25–30 minutes, until firm to the touch and golden on top. Cool the muffins for 2–3 minutes and serve them warm or at room temperature.

Green tea bread serves 6

CIRCULATORY

375g (12oz) seedless raisins
    and sultanas, mixed
300ml (½pt) green tea (or
    your favourite tea)
175g (6oz) soft brown sugar
250g (8oz) wholemeal
    self-raising flour
1 egg
1tsp mixed spice
grated zest of 1 lemon
90g (3oz) mixed chopped
    almonds, walnuts, and
    hazelnuts

Put the dried fruit in a large bowl and stir in the tea and sugar. Cover and set aside to soak overnight. Next day, preheat the oven to 180°C (350°F/gas 4). Lightly grease a 1kg (2lb) loaf tin. Add the remaining ingredients to the dried-fruit mixture and beat well. Pour into the prepared loaf tin, pushing the mixture into the corners of the tin. Transfer to the preheated oven and bake for 1 hour 15 minutes, or until a skewer inserted into the centre of the bread comes out clean. Turn out of the tin and leave to cool on a wire rack.

Blueberry muffins serves 6

CIRCULATORY · DIGESTIVE · FATIGUE

100g (3½oz) self raising flour
60g (2oz) wholemeal flour
1 tsp baking powder
1 tsp mixed spice
125ml (4fl oz) milk
60g (2oz) butter, melted
1 large egg
2tsp lemon juice
90g (3oz) soft brown sugar
90g (3oz) fresh blueberries

Preheat the oven to 180°C (350°F/gas 4). Put 12 paper muffin cases into a muffin tin. Sift the flours, baking powder, and mixed spice into a mixing bowl, putting the bran in the sieve back into the bowl. Beat together the milk, butter, egg, lemon juice, and sugar in a bowl or wide jug. Make a well in the centre of the flour mixture and pour in half the milk mixture. Gently fold it in, then add the rest and stir it in. Fold in the blueberries.

Spoon the mixture into the muffin cases and bake in the oven for about 20 minutes, until well risen and golden on top. Take the muffins out of the tin and leave on a wire rack to cool.

Banana and walnut bread serves 6

CIRCULATORY · DIGESTIVE · FATIGUE

250g (8oz) cottage cheese,
    pressed through a sieve
125g (4oz) soft brown sugar
3 eggs, beaten
60g (2oz) chopped walnuts
2 bananas, mashed
250g (8oz) wholemeal
    self-raising flour

Preheat the oven to 180°C (350°F/gas 4). Line a 1kg (2lb) loaf tin with greased greaseproof paper or baking parchment. Cream the cottage cheese and sugar together until well blended. Gradually beat in the eggs. Add the chopped nuts and bananas and mix well. Add the flour, mixing it in well. Spoon the mixture into the prepared tin, pressing it into the corners. Bake in the oven for 40–45 minutes, or until a skewer inserted into the centre of the bread comes out clean. Cool on a wire rack and serve in lightly buttered slices.

Avocado and watercress salad serves 4 ▶

CANCER · CIRCULATORY · STRESS · FATIGUE · SKIN

1 bunch watercress
2 avocados
30g (1oz) pine nuts
2tbs walnut oil
juice of half a lemon
salt and pepper

Wash and dry the watercress, discard the bigger stalks, and put the cress in a salad bowl. Add the avocados, sliced thinly, and the pine nuts. Make a dressing with the walnut oil, lemon juice, salt, and pepper and pour over. Toss very gently, then chill, covered with a damp cloth, for an hour or so before eating.

Red bean salad in plum sauce serves 4

CANCER · CIRCULATORY · STRESS · SKIN

1 clove garlic
dash cayenne pepper
6 leaves fresh basil, torn
    in pieces
a few sprigs of fresh
    coriander
1tbs red wine vinegar
5tbs damson jam
1tbs olive oil
375g (12oz) cooked red
kidney
    beans, drained

Nathalie Hambro gives the recipe for this piquant salad in her book *Particular Delights*. Although it sounds a little strange, this traditional dish from the country of Georgia is a real taste-treat.

Crush the garlic. Add the cayenne, basil, and some of the coriander leaves, chopped, and mash the mixture to a smooth paste. Combine the vinegar and jam in an enamel or stainless-steel pan and boil over a high heat, stirring constantly, until the jam is dissolved. Rub the mixture through a fine sieve, add the oil, then gradually beat it into the garlic and herb paste. Add the beans and toss gently but thoroughly. Cover and refrigerate overnight. Serve decorated with the remaining coriander leaves.

Tomato salad serves 4

CANCER · CIRCULATORY · DIGESTIVE · FATIGUE

4 tomatoes
4 cloves garlic, finely chopped
2tbs fresh basil, chives, or
    parsley, finely chopped
2tbs spring onions, chopped
sea salt and freshly ground
    black pepper
2tbs extra-virgin olive oil

Slice the tomatoes finely. Arrange them on a serving dish. Clean, trim, and chop the spring onions. Strew the chopped garlic across the tomatoes, top with the chopped green herbs and the chopped spring onions, add a little freshly ground pepper and a touch of salt, and drizzle the oil over the surface.

Waldorf salad serves 4

CANCER · CIRCULATORY · DIGESTIVE · JOINTS · RESPIRATORY

4 sticks celery
2 large eating apples
a handful of raisins
1tbs olive oil
1tsp lemon juice
150g (5oz) natural yoghurt
salt and pepper
1tbs parsley, finely chopped
60g (2oz) walnuts

Clean and slice the celery into small chunks; wash and core the apples and cut into small slices; wash and dry the raisins. Put celery, apple chunks, and raisins into a salad bowl. Stir the olive oil and lemon juice into the yoghurt, season with salt and pepper, and add to the salad. Toss lightly and garnish with the walnuts and parsley.

Complete coleslaw serves 4

CANCER · CIRCULATORY · DIGESTIVE · FATIGUE · JOINTS

half small white cabbage
2 carrots
1 small eating apple
juice of half a lemon
1tbs olive oil
150g (5oz) natural yoghurt
salt, pepper, and fresh chervil

Wash and shred the cabbage, wash and grate the carrots, and wash and shred the apple, and then put them all in a salad bowl. Sprinkle with the lemon juice. Stir the oil into the yoghurt, season with salt and pepper to taste, and stir into the slaw. Cover and chill for at least an hour. Garnish with chopped chervil before serving.

Celery, radish, and walnut salad serves 4

CANCER · DIGESTIVE · STRESS · JOINTS · SKIN

1 bunch radishes
3–4 sticks celery
125g (4oz) walnuts
2tbs extra-virgin olive oil
1tsp lemon juice
salt and pepper

Scrub the radishes and cut into fine slices; save the best unwilted bits of the green leafy tops. Clean the celery and slice finely; save some of the feathery fronds. Roughly chop the walnuts. Make a dressing with the oil, lemon, and salt and pepper to taste. Stir thoroughly. Arrange the celery, radishes, and walnuts on a flat dish. Spoon the dressing over and decorate with the radish and celery fronds.

Winter white salad serves 4

CANCER · CIRCULATORY · STRESS · FATIGUE · JOINTS

1 large fennel bulb
a chunk crisp white cabbage
2 sticks celery
2–3 white radishes
2tbs oil
1tbs lemon juice
salt and pepper
1tbs fresh parsley,
   finely chopped

Clean and slice the fennel into strips, saving the feathery fronds; clean and shred the cabbage; clean and slice the celery; clean and slice the radishes. Arrange in the salad bowl. In a separate bowl, mix the oil, lemon juice, and salt and pepper, and pour over. Toss. Garnish with the parsley.

Apricot whip serves 4

CANCER · CIRCULATORY · DIGESTIVE · FATIGUE · JOINTS

250g (8oz) dried apricots
300ml (½pt) water
1tbs apple juice concentrate
1tbs lemon juice
1–2tbs honey
4tbs Greek yoghurt
¼tsp nutmeg
1tbs flaked almonds

Wash the apricots. Mix the water with the apple juice concentrate, lemon juice, and honey. Pour the mixture over the apricots and leave to soak, covered, overnight. Next day, put the apricots in a pan with the liquid, bring to the boil, and simmer until soft – about 5–10 minutes. Leave to cool, then purée. Spoon into individual glass dishes; top with a spoonful of Greek yoghurt, a dusting of nutmeg, and a few flaked almonds.

Spiced peaches serves 4 ▶

DIGESTIVE · STRESS · FATIGUE · RESPIRATORY · SKIN

8 small peaches
8 cloves
enough red or white wine
    to cover
peel of 1 lemon
1tbs honey
¼tsp nutmeg or cinnamon

A clever cook we know invented this all-purpose pudding on holiday in Spain, profiting by a glut of tiny peaches at give-away prices and cheap local wine. It is highly adaptable; we have cooked hard little apricots or nectarines the same way, or used up oddments of brandy, whisky, apple, or grape juice instead. Chilled and piled up in a dish with the syrupy remains of the juice poured over, and with Greek yoghurt or cream served separately, it can be a grand party pudding. Any leftovers never survive breakfast time.

Wash the peaches, stick a clove in each one, and put in a pan with the wine. Add the peel of a well-scrubbed lemon, honey, and nutmeg or cinnamon to taste. Bring to the boil, lower the heat, and simmer, covered, until the peaches are tender and almost at bursting point.

Mont blanc serves 4

CIRCULATORY · FATIGUE

500g (1lb) tin of unsweetened
    chestnut purée
1tbs brown sugar
rind and juice of 1 orange
6tbs thick cream or
    crème fraîche
1tbs bitter chocolate, grated,
    to garnish

Put the chestnut purée, sugar, and orange juice and rind in a food processor and blend until smooth. Add 4 tablespoons of the cream or crème fraîche and blend again. Serve heaped in a mound on a pretty dish, topped with the rest of the cream or crème fraîche, and sprinkle the grated chocolate on top.

Red plum pudding serves 4

CIRCULATORY · DIGESTIVE

500g (1lb) dark red plums,
    washed and stoned
2tsp runny honey
2tbs red wine
4–6 cardamom pods
1tbs cassis or brandy

Put the plums in a pan with the honey, the wine, and the cardamom pods. Simmer over a low heat until the plums are just starting to disintegrate, then add the brandy (alcohol, incidentally, evaporates when heated, leaving only the flavour behind). Heat through again and transfer to a serving dish. Serve with cream, yoghurt, fromage frais, or crème fraîche. This pudding is also delicious served cold.

Crowdie serves 4

STRESS · FATIGUE

125g (4oz) coarse oats
60g (2oz) flaked almonds
1tbs brown sugar
250g (8oz) whipping cream
250g (8oz) Greek yoghurt

Spread the oats and flaked almonds on a flat baking tray and sprinkle with the sugar. Place in a hot oven until crispy but not browned. Reserve one tablespoon of this mixture. Whip the cream, fold in the yoghurt, stir in the oat-and-almond mixture, and spoon into glass dishes. Decorate with the reserved oats and almond mix.

Spicy winter pudding serves 4

CANCER · DIGESTIVE · FATIGUE · RESPIRATORY

300ml (½pt) apple juice
4 cloves
a little freshly grated ginger,
    or ½tsp powdered ginger
½tsp cinnamon
good pinch grated nutmeg
1tbs honey
250g (8oz) assorted stoned or
    seedless dried fruit
    – prunes, apricots, raisins,
    apples, pears, washed
twist of lemon peel
8–10 pieces wholewheat
    bread, thinly sliced and
    lightly buttered

Heat up the apple juice with the cloves, ginger, cinnamon, nutmeg, and honey. When it is boiling, add the fruit and the lemon peel and simmer very gently for about 25 minutes or until the fruit is soft. Drain, saving the juices. Meanwhile, grease a heatproof dish, then line with thin slices of wholewheat bread, crusts removed. Fill with the fruit mixture, top with more bread, and pour over it enough of the cooking liquid to saturate the bread. Sprinkle the top with a little brown sugar and cinnamon. Put in a moderate oven for 20–25 minutes. Pour the remaining cooking liquid over it.

Blackcurrant jelly serves 4

DIGESTIVE · FATIGUE · RESPIRATORY

1kg (2lb) blackcurrants
600ml (1pt) apple juice
2tsp agar-agar
small red eating apple
honey to taste

Wash and trim the blackcurrants. Heat the apple juice, add the agar-agar, and bring gently to the boil, stirring until all the agar-agar is dissolved. Mix with the blackcurrants, wet a jelly mould, pour all the mixture in, and place in the refrigerator. When just beginning to set, core the apple and cut it into fine slices. Arrange on the half-set jelly and return to the refrigerator until set.

Vegetable stock serves 4

DIGESTIVE · FATIGUE · JOINTS · RESPIRATORY

2 large carrots
1 large onion
2-3 cloves garlic
2 sticks celery, including tops
2tbs olive oil
1 bay leaf
1tbs each fresh thyme and
   marjoram, chopped
900ml (1½pt) water

Peel and slice the carrots, peel and chop the onion and garlic, and clean and chop the celery. Heat the oil in a big saucepan, melt the onion and garlic, add the carrot and celery, stir and cook gently for about 5 minutes. Add the herbs and water, bring to the boil, and simmer for about an hour, covered.

Wholemeal garlic croutons serves 4

STRESS · FATIGUE · RESPIRATORY

2 thick slices wholemeal
   bread – not too fresh
2tbs olive oil
2 cloves garlic, crushed

Add the crushed garlic to the oil and leave for at least an hour. Then cut and discard the bread-crusts, cut the slices into cubes, strain the olive oil into a baking dish, turn the cubes into it and turn them around in the garlicky oil. Bake in a hot oven until they are crispy brown – about 20 minutes. For plain wholemeal croutons, simply omit the garlic.

Basic barley serves 4

CIRCULATORY · DIGESTIVE · FATIGUE · URINARY

250g (8oz) pot barley
750ml (1¼pt) water

Wash the barley thoroughly. Put it in a pan with the water and bring to the boil. Lower the heat and simmer, covered, for 45 minutes, or until the barley is tender. Drain the barley, but don't throw away the water: it is nutritionally rich. Add to soups or stews, or drink it on its own.

Tomato sauce serves 4

CANCER · CIRCULATORY

2tbs olive oil
2 cloves garlic, finely chopped
1 medium-sized onion, chopped
2 425g (14oz) tins of Italian plum tomatoes
salt and pepper
2tbs fresh parsley, chopped

Heat the oil, put in the finely chopped garlic and onion, and fry gently without browning. Add the tomatoes and their juice and cook briskly, uncovered, stirring occasionally, for about 20 minutes. When the sauce thickens, purée it in a blender or food processor, reheat, season with salt and pepper to taste, and stir in the parsley.

Serve with plain grilled fish, meat, or pasta. Add a small finely chopped chilli pepper or a half a teaspoon cayenne pepper and this becomes the traditionally fiery arrabbiata literally "raging" – tomato sauce beloved of the Italians, and served with pasta – usually the big tubes of penne. It goes superbly with any dried pasta.

Index

★★★★

index 191

Acknowledgments

★★★★

ABOUT THE AUTHORS
One of the leading authorities on complementary health, Michael van Straten is a former president of the British Naturopathic and Osteopathic Association and a past governor of the British College of Naturopathy and Osteopathy. A practising osteopath, naturopath, acupuncturist, and nutritional consultant and a well-known medical broadcaster and writer, he also contributes regularly to television shows.

Michael has more than 20 health titles to his name, including the best-selling books from DK's *Superfoods* series, and the phenomenally successful *Foods That Harm, Foods That Heal*, for which he was a Consultant Editor. A colourful personality and an enthusiastic cook, his hobby is making jams and chutneys from the produce he grows on his organic farm.

He relieves stress by beating dough during his weekend bread making sessions.

Barbara Griggs has been researching, writing, and lecturing about health and herbal medicine for more than 30 years. She is the author of a number of books on nutrition and herbal medicine, and as a journalist she is well known for the articles she contributed regularly to *Country Living*, where she was Health Editor for 20 years.

PUBLISHER'S ACKNOWLEDGMENTS
Dorling Kindersley would like to thank Sîan Irvine for photography; home economist Pippin Britz; Alyson Lacewing, Katie John, and Helen Murray for editorial assistance; Iona Hoyle for design assistance; Christine Heilman and Jennifer Williams for editing the North American edition, and Marie Lorimer for compiling the index.

★★

AUTHORS' ACKNOWLEDGMENTS
The authors would like to thank the DK team for all their hard work, especially: editors, Shannon Beatty and Kathy Fahey and designers, Anne Fisher and Ruth Hope. They would also like to thank the following authors and publishers for their permission to quote excerpts from their work:

Marcella Hazan (White bean soup) from *Essentials of Classic Italian Cooking* (Macmillan London Ltd.); Rosemary Man and Robin Weir (Devilled chicken) from *The Compleat Mustard* (Constable); Pat Chapman (Chicken jalfrezi) from *Favourite Restaurant Curries* (Judy Piatkus Publishers); Paul

Laurenson and Ethel Minogue (Falafel) from *The Taste of Health* (BBC Books); Nathalie Hambro (Red bean salad in plum sauce) from *Particular Delights* (Ebury). They would also like to thank J. Sainsbury plc for permission to reproduce a recipe (Peppered fish with vinaigrette) from one of their leaflets.

Some text from the Superfoods section first appeared in *Superfeast* by Michael van Straten published in 2005 by Little Books, Inc. and is reproduced by kind permission of the publisher.

PICTURE CREDITS
All images © DK Images